CONSUMERGUIDE®

Foods that Make You Lose Weight

FAT-FIGHTING FOODS FOR A HEALTHIER YOU

Gayle Alleman, M.S., R.D.
Susan Male Smith, M.A., R.D.
Densie Webb, Ph.D., R.D.

 Publications International, Ltd.

Contributing Writers

Gayle Alleman, M.S., R.D., holds degrees in both alternative and conventional nutrition. She manages the nutrition education program for Washington State University Cooperative Extension and teaches nutrition at Bastyr University and other colleges. She is also a freelance writer and speaker in the area of food, nutrition, and health, specializing in holistic nutrition to promote optimum health.

Susan Male Smith, M.A., R.D., is a registered dietitian and nutrition consultant who writes for such consumer magazines as *Family Circle, Redbook, McCall's, American Health,* and *Baby Talk.* In 1994, she was nominated for a James Beard Journalism Award. Ms. Smith is assistant editor of *Environmental Nutrition* newsletter.

Densie Webb, Ph.D., R.D., is a nutrition writer and registered dietitian. She is editor of *Environmental Nutrition* newsletter and has written several nutritional analysis books. She also contributes to consumer magazines such as *American Health, Woman's Day,* and *Family Circle.* Dr. Webb has also served as health editor of *McCall's* magazine.

Cover photo credit: **R. Pleasant/FPG International**

Louis Weber, CEO
Publications International, Ltd.
7373 North Cicero Avenue
Lincolnwood, Illinois 60712

Permission is never granted for commercial purposes.

ISBN 13: 978-0-7853-3373-9
ISBN 10: 0-7853-3373-8

Manufactured in U.S.A.

8 7 6 5 4 3 2 1

CONTENTS

Contents

INTRODUCTION

By opening this book, you must be ready to lose weight. Congratulations! That decision will mean a healthier you, and we will help you get there. By dropping those extra pounds and keeping them off, you'll not only feel better and more energetic, you'll also lower your risk of health problems such as heart disease, diabetes, and certain cancers. And the best part is, the foods you'll be eating are delicious and filling.

In the search for the "perfect" diet, there are many choices. The most successful ones are not diets at all, but actually new ways of eating that become a part of your normal lifestyle. You can lose weight easily—almost magically—when you enjoy foods that promote weight loss by their very nature: foods that are low in calories and fat and rich in fiber and nutrients. This book will show you how to use those foods to make tasty and satisfying meals.

Don't be fooled by diet schemes that make unrealistic demands such as drinking a liquid diet, focusing on one food group, fasting or starving yourself, or requiring unbalanced meal plans. To succeed at long-term weight loss, it's important to learn new ways of eating that you enjoy enough to continue doing. If you "diet" for awhile, restricting whatever foods the current fad diet suggests, but then return to your old eating habits, the weight will come crashing back on—just what you don't want.

The best plan for achieving a healthy weight and maintaining it is to gradually change the foods you eat. This book will help you do just that! The food profiles that appear later will show you how to choose foods that can help you get trim. The profiles also provide tips on how to select and prepare these fat-fighting foods. There's no gimmick about them—they're chock-full of satisfying complex carbohydrates, brimming with fiber to give you a feeling of fullness, and rich in nutrients to keep you naturally healthy, so your body doesn't crave more food than it needs. Let's discover just how these wonder foods do this.

A DIET THAT'S MORE THAN SKIN DEEP

Compared to the standard American diet, the eating plan you are about to embark on is much healthier. It encourages you to eat a variety of complex carbohydrates such as fruits, vegetables, legumes, and whole grains with a few dairy and protein foods to keep your body in tip-top shape. You'll get full enough on these foods that you won't feel the need to reach for those boxes and packages of processed crackers, cookies,

---

HEALTHY SIDE EFFECTS

By basing your diet on the foods in this book, you can lose weight AND:

Lessen your chances of heart disease, heart attack, and stroke

Reduce your risk of colon cancer

Lower your blood cholesterol levels

Lessen your chance of developing adult-onset diabetes

Get all the benefits of disease-fighting phytochemicals

---

and snack foods. This not only makes it easier to keep calories under control, but your wallet will appreciate it, too. Processed foods are expensive; the natural, whole foods in this book are not. So you end up trimming your waistline while fattening your wallet at the same time.

For years, researchers have noticed that people who eat less meat or who are vegetarian are not only slimmer than their meat-eating counterparts, they also have a lower incidence of heart disease, heart attacks, and stroke. The eating strategies in this book will let you enjoy these health benefits too, since the plan is primarily vegetarian with the inclusion of fish and low-fat dairy products. Fish provides heart-healthy omega-3 fatty acids, which will be discussed in detail shortly.

The fiber in these foods will not only provide satiety and quell your appetite, they will also fight colon cancer at the same time. Standard American fare, which is usually very low in fiber, is linked to many intestinal disorders, such as diverticulosis and colon cancer. Studies repeatedly show that people who eat more fiber, especially the insoluble type, have a lower incidence of colon cancer. So as you embark on this high-fiber eating plan, you're protecting your colon, too.

The other kind of fiber, soluble fiber, lowers blood cholesterol. As you enjoy the foods in this book, you'll be driving your cholesterol level down and protecting your blood vessels and heart. In fact, this eating plan can help reverse clogged arteries, as you eat more soluble fiber each day.

Both kinds of fiber help to slow the absorption of sugars—natural or added—which means they help stabilize blood glucose levels. A carefully monitored, fiber-rich diet is sometimes enough to enable a person with diabetes who only takes oral

THE FACES OF FIBER

Insoluble Fiber: This is what you traditionally think of as fiber—as in bran cereal and bran muffins. This kind of fiber can be likened to a sponge. When you eat fiber then add water, it swells and gets soft, just like a sponge. The increased bulk pushes on your intestines, creating the rhythmic movement needed to evacuate. And a softer stool is easier on your intestines. Foods rich in insoluble fiber include bran cereals, brown rice, corn and popcorn, fruits (especially apples, berries, and pears), whole grains, and vegetables (especially asparagus, kale, peas, potatoes, and spinach).

Soluble Fiber: This is the gummy stuff that gunks up the works. But that's its job. As its name suggests, soluble fiber dissolves in water. In doing so, it forms a gel-like substance, which captures bile acids and cholesterol in its wake. Foods rich in soluble fiber include barley, dried beans and peas, fruits (especially apples, figs, oranges, plums, and rhubarb), lentils, oats, and vegetables (especially broccoli, cabbage, carrots, okra, and potatoes).

medication to stop doing so. Dropping extra pounds can prevent or even reverse adult-onset diabetes.

Phytochemicals are "plant chemicals," substances that a plant naturally makes that happen to be beneficial to those who eat them. Many phytochemicals are antioxidants, which help protect cells from cancer, protect blood vessels from tiny injuries that start atherosclerosis, and protect eyes from developing cataracts. Other phytochemicals help boost immune function and still others improve the health and integrity of your blood vessels. A plant-based diet is rich in phytochemicals.

STOP THE DIETING

Repeated weight loss and gain carries health risks that you don't need, such as a greater likelihood of heart disease than if you had never lost weight at all. And as you may have heard, it is harder to lose weight each time you do it. Here's why: If your "diet" includes skipping meals, fasting, or eating less than 1,000 calories per day, it lowers your body's metabolic rate. The metabolic rate is the amount of energy, or calories, a resting, awake body needs just to breathe and stay alive. If you don't eat on a regular basis or eat too little, the body thinks it's starving, so it begins to shut down and conserve resources. This is part of the human body's evolutionary design, slowing down to survive periods when food is scarce. Your body doesn't know you're dieting; it thinks the world is on the brink of a famine, so it switches into "starvation mode" to conserve fat stores. The lower your metabolic rate goes, the more difficult it is to lose weight. In fact, just skipping breakfast every day lowers your metabolic rate by four to five percent, resulting in a one-pound weight gain every seven weeks without eating any extra food.

To make matters worse, when this process happens, your body hangs on tightly to its fat stores, because those are concentrated sources of energy it might need if the famine lasts a long time. So instead, it sacrifices protein from your muscles to make the energy it needs. As you lose muscle—the body's main energy burner—your metabolic rate drops even lower, beginning a downward spiral. What you want to do instead is preserve lean muscle tissue, because it has a higher metabolic rate, and get rid of fat tissue, which has a low metabolic rate.

To prevent your body from switching into this "starvation mode" and burning up muscle, you need to eat at least 1,200 calories per day divided up into at least three meals. You'll probably need to eat about 1,200 to 1,800 calories, depending on your size and sex, to get all the vitamins and minerals you need and not feel hungry or deprived.

Many people try to diet by purchasing nonfat convenience foods and snack foods. Never before have there been so many nonfat or reduced-fat products in the supermarket, yet the rate of overweight and obesity in America is at an all-time high. This is due in part to the plethora of non- and low-fat foods that are stripped of their fiber and loaded with sugar and, consequently, calories. These simple carbohydrates, or sugars, give you calories but few nutrients—what you want instead are complex carbohydrates, which are starches. It's much better to eat nature's low-calorie foods, such as grains, vegetables, legumes, and fruits, than to fill up on sugar-laden, fiber-deficient processed foods.

Some popular diet plans advocate eating large amounts of protein and quite a bit of fat while reducing calories overall. It's the calorie reduction that makes these plans work...for a little while. Plus the fact that since your body is starving for carbohydrates, it is forced to break down muscle, which has a considerable amount of water in it. It's usually not long before the dieter gets so tired of the limited foods that they "fall off the wagon" and go back to their old eating habits.

A high-protein diet can carry other risks with it, too. Excessive amounts of protein on a daily basis can cause dehydration, tax the kidneys, and send you into ketosis—a condition in which your body is struggling to make the carbohydrates it needs for energy since you aren't eating enough of them. Ketosis can upset the body's delicate pH balance, and if severe enough, it can lead to coma and even death. Carbohydrates are the clean fuel your body's engine wants to burn; protein is like dirty fuel that can gum up your engine.

Your body needs carbohydrates not only to provide you with energy to walk, think, problem solve, love, play, and do all your daily activities, but also to burn up fat. The body must have some carbohydrates to combine with the fat being released from fat cells in order to turn that fat into energy. It's this simple:

Fat + carbohydrates = energy

Fat with no carbohydrates = dangerous ketones

Most diet plans are strict regimes that don't let you experience making healthy food choices for yourself. Learning and practicing new eating behaviors is the only way you'll be able to maintain weight loss.

SHED POUNDS THIS WAY

So the best way to get rid of fat cells is to pump your body full of unrefined, complex carbohydrates, add a little protein and fat, and mix with physical activity. It's the perfect recipe for weight loss, and the eating plan and foods in this book will help you do just that. You'll get not only plenty of carbohydrates, but you'll learn how to combine them to get good quality protein, plus a little fish for those heart-healthy omega-3 fatty acids, and a few servings of skim milk or non-fat yogurt every day to keep your bones rich in calcium.

The recently revised U.S. Department of Agriculture (USDA) Dietary Guidelines for Americans (2005) promote just this type of eating. And for the first time, the Guidelines emphasize weight loss in addition to nutritional advice.

The new dietary recommendations include an increased intake of fruits and vegetables (4.5 cups per day) to fill you up on fewer calories and increase your fiber intake, and an additional serving of low-fat or nonfat dairy (3 cups per day), because studies show consuming that amount of dairy, along with a healthy eating and activity plan, may improve weight loss. The Guidelines also recommend that half your daily intake (6 ounces) of grains come from whole grains, which also contain lots of fiber to fill you up and not out.

Accompanying the Guidelines is a new symbol called My-Pyramid that replaces the original Food Guide Pyramid. As you can see on the next page, the new pyramid emphasizes the importance of getting daily physical activity, as well as making smart food choices from each food group every day. MyPyramid is deliberately simple in design to reflect the need for an individualized approach to diet and physical activity.

Here's the number of servings we recommend for weight loss. Make sure the serving sizes are no larger than what the Dietary Guidelines recommend (see "What Is a Serving?," page 15).

Breads, Cereals, Pasta	6 servings
Vegetables	3–4 servings
Fruits	2 servings
Dairy products (nonfat)	2 servings
Fish or protein foods	2 servings

Here's one way to put these servings together to get a balanced, weight-reduction meal plan every day. It provides you with a lot of flexibility to choose the foods that you like and as much or as little variety as you enjoy.

Breakfast—Eat breakfast within two hours of getting up, every day, to get your metabolism revved up. As you choose foods from each of these groups, make sure your choices are low in fat and added sugar.

1   bread, cereal, or grain (such as toast or cereal)

1   fruit (such as 1 piece or ½ cup of juice)

1   dairy (such as nonfat milk or sugar-free nonfat yogurt)

Snack—Eat one serving of a low-fat, low-sugar bread, cereal, or grain (such as ½ bagel).

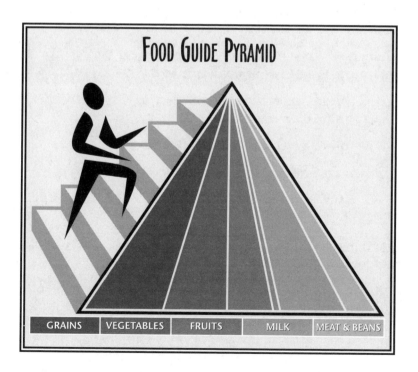

FOOD GUIDE PYRAMID

| GRAINS | VEGETABLES | FRUITS | MILK | MEAT & BEANS |

Lunch—Eat one or two servings from these food groups, as indicated. Make low- or nonfat choices.

2 bread, cereal, or grain (such as a sandwich or tortillas)

1 protein (such as baked fish or beans)

2 vegetable (lettuce and tomato on sandwich or in tortilla, carrot sticks)

1 fruit (or save until dinner)

1 dairy (or save until afternoon snack)

Snack—Eat one serving of a low-fat, low-sugar bread, cereal, or grain (such as reduced-fat graham crackers) or save until dinner. Have one serving of nonfat or low-fat dairy.

Dinner—Eat one or two servings from these food groups, as indicated. Make low- or nonfat choices.

1 or 2 breads, cereals, or grain (2 servings if you saved one from afternoon snack)

1 protein (such as spicy black beans)

2 vegetable (such as steamed vegetable and salad)

1 fruit (if saved from lunch; try a baked apple or pear for dessert)

Snack—Don't do it. Brush your teeth instead. The sweetness of toothpaste often alleviates late-evening cravings.

You can mix these categories around if you like, as long as you don't exceed the total number of recommended servings. Keep in mind your metabolism will run at a higher rate if you eat several small meals and snacks throughout the day,

WHAT IS A SERVING?

To end consumer confusion over what constitutes a serving, the new Dietary Guidelines describe servings in familiar household measurements, such as cups and ounces. The new guidelines tell you exactly how much food you should be taking in from each food group, while the old guidelines just recommended a number of servings per food group without describing what that meant. The new Guidelines take the guesswork out of meal planning and better help you meet your diet and weight-loss goals. The following are equivalents to the quantities recommended in the Guidelines.

Grains. *One ounce-equivalent is the same as*
1 slice bread
1 cup cereal flakes
½ cup cooked rice, pasta, or cereal
1 ounce dry pasta or rice
1 very small muffin (1 ounce)

Vegetables and fruits. *One-half cup fruit or vegetables is equivalent to*
½ cup of cut-up raw or cooked fruit or vegetable
½ cup fruit or vegetable juice
1 cup raw, leafy salad greens
Meat and Beans *One ounce-equivalent is the same as*
1 ounce lean meat, poultry, or fish

1 egg
¼ cup cooked dry beans or tofu (count as vegetable or protein, not both)
1 tablespoon peanut butter
½ ounce nuts or seeds

Milk. *One cup milk is equivalent to*
1 cup milk, yogurt, or fortified soy milk
1½ ounces natural cheese
2 ounces processed cheese

Oils. *One teaspoon is equivalent to*
1 teaspoon soft margarine
1 tablespoon low-fat mayonnaise
2 tablespoons light salad dressing

TRICKS OF THE TRADE

Use some of the following tried-and-true tips to enhance your new eating style and make it even more effective for you:

Shop when you're not hungry.

Store tempting foods out of sight; leave preferred foods in sight.

Use smaller plates and bowls.

Set your fork down between bites.

Chew thoroughly and swallow before taking another bite.

Eat mindfully, not in front of the TV or while reading.

Twice a week, write down everything you eat and drink in a 24-hour period. Does it match your plan and goal for number of servings from each group?

Plan nonfood rewards for following your new eating style.

instead of going for long periods of time without food, making your body wonder if starvation is imminent. Learn to listen to your body's cues; eat when you're hungry without putting it off. If you're not hungry between meals, skip the snacks and add those portions in somewhere else. It's better to eat the majority of your food earlier in the day, rather than close to bedtime, so that it is processed before you go to sleep.

Prepare complex carbohydrates in ways that are tasty to you. Check the food profile pages for new ideas. You'll lose interest in your new eating plan if you don't like the way your food tastes.

Benefits of Carbohydrates

Complex carbohydrates, such as those found in whole grains, legumes, fruits, and vegetables, help to jump-start your metabolism. A number of research studies using both animals and people show that a high-carbohydrate diet boosts T_3 levels. In fact, some research indicates that carbohydrates are a very important regulator of T_3 production in humans. T_3 is a thyroid hormone that's responsible for revving up the body's base metabolic rate. There's also some scientific evidence that carbohydrates boost your body's production of norepinephrine. Norepinephrine is another hormone that stimulates metabolic rate. So by eating complex carbohydrates, you can help prevent your metabolism from becoming sluggish. Exercise works much the same way, but you'll learn more about that later.

One of the major benefits of complex carbohydrates is that they're naturally low in calories. Carbohydrates have only four calories per gram. Compare that to the nine calories in every gram of fat and you begin to get the picture. See for yourself in this chart that shows the amount of calories found in a typical serving, versus the amount of calories in a processed form of the food:

Fruit (1 piece)	60 calories	Fruit pie (1 piece)	300 calories
Vegetables (½ cup raw)	25 calories	Potato chips (20)	215 calories
Bread (1 slice)	80 calories	Glazed doughnut	242 calories
Legumes (½ cup)	115 calories	Ground beef patty	250 calories

Of course, what you put on your carbohydrates makes a difference, too. If you add sauces full of butter, cream, or cheese, that's going to drastically increase the calorie count. If you slather butter onto your bread or baked potato or douse your salad with an oily or creamy dressing, that, too, will ruin the low-calorie benefit of those foods. Likewise, turning your fruit into pie will dramatically change its calorie count for the worse. Instead, just follow the serving suggestions listed in the food profile section to help you enjoy the true taste of foods such as juicy pineapple, sweet corn, fresh baked whole-wheat bread, and spicy bean dishes.

Another exciting benefit of eating complex carbohydrates is that you automatically boost your fiber intake. It is recommended that everyone eat 20 to 35 grams of fiber each day. You'll want to aim for the higher end of that range. Fiber is especially helpful when you're trying to lose weight because it helps you feel full, so you don't overeat. Fiber slows the rate at which your stomach empties and takes a while to work its way through your digestive system. It also enables the sugars in your meal to be absorbed slowly. Both of these feats help that feeling of fullness last just a little longer, which, in turn, means your appetite is delayed; you don't feel hungry again so soon. Don't fret too much about overdoing fiber. It takes more than 75 grams per day before adverse effects set in, and it's hard to eat that much fiber.

It's absolutely essential that as you begin to eat more fiber-rich complex carbohydrates, you also begin to drink more water. Without enough fluid, the extra fiber will backfire on you and make you gassy and constipated. Drink at least six 8-ounce glasses of water every day, and drink other beverages, too. Coffee and black tea don't count since they have diuretic properties, making you lose water.

A CALORIE IS A CALORIE—OR IS IT?

One of the secrets behind eating a diet rich in complex carbohydrates is that the body processes carbohydrates differently than it processes fat. It's easy for the body to break down fat, absorb it, and store it. Nature arranged for the body to store fat without much ado, so that it has plenty of stored energy in case of unexpected scarcity or famine.

Carbohydrates and protein, on the other hand, are more difficult for the body to break down, absorb, process, store, and use. It's a much more complicated chemical process to get energy out of carbohydrates and protein than it is to get energy from fat.

As we've mentioned, fat contains nine calories per gram, whereas carbohydrates and protein each contain only four calories per gram. But some scientists wonder whether these numbers should be adjusted. Since it doesn't take much energy for the body to use fat, researchers speculate that it may actually have a caloric value that is closer to eleven calories per gram. And because carbohydrates take a lot of energy to process, their true caloric value might be closer to three calories per gram. Although the official numbers have not been changed yet, the underlying principal still remains: A diet that is high in complex carbohydrates, low in fat, and accompanied by some protein can help you shed unwanted pounds.

Here's an example to illustrate how this works. When you eat 100 calories of carbohydrates, you only get about 74 calories out of that food by the time the body processes it. In other words, it takes 26 calories to process that 100 calories you ate. On the other hand, when you eat 100 calories of fat, you get about 97 calories by the time the body processes it; it takes only 3 calories to process 100 grams of fat. Quite a difference, isn't it? That's why fat makes you fat; it's not only concentrated, carrying more than twice the amount of calories as carbohydrates, it doesn't take much work or energy for the body to process it. It's a simple matter of math: The more carbohydrates and less fat you eat, the fewer calories you'll have to add to your waistline.

IS THE "NEGATIVE CALORIE EFFECT" TRUE?

Generally speaking, nutrition experts say that the body uses about ten percent of all the calories it consumes just to process food. This is called the thermic effect of food. In light of the previous discussion, we see how this rate can get bumped up. By eating more carbohydrates and less fat, the thermic effect of our meal will be more than ten percent. So this is how the negative calorie effect works. Complex carbohydrates take nearly 25 percent of the energy they give just to be processed.

Some people believe that the "negative calorie effect" means that you'll spend more energy eating and processing a food than you'll get from it. This isn't quite true because you'll always spend just a percentage of the total carbohydrates you eat on processing them. The fallacy comes from the fact that some very-low-calorie foods may come close to that. For instance, one cup of chopped romaine lettuce has 9 calories, mostly from carbohydrates, but you'll net only 6.75 calories from it. Close to zero, but not quite, and certainly not a negative number.

MODERATION IN ALL THINGS

Besides filling up on complex carbohydrates, it's important to make low-fat choices. Foods high in fat, such as nuts or avocados, should be eaten only occasionally; eat high-fat snack foods only rarely.

In your zeal to lose weight, keep in mind that you need some fat each day, and not all fats are bad. In fact, the body has to have dietary fat to provide you with the essential fatty acids that cannot be made inside the body. Without essential fatty acids, skin may become dry, cholesterol and triglycerides in the blood may skyrocket, and blood pressure may rise. Essential fatty acids help your body make substances called prostaglandins that keep all these processes in balance.

Fat in the diet is also the only way we get the essential fat soluble vitamins A, E, and K. The body cannot make these vitamins, so they must come from the diet.

The minimum amount of fat recommended in the diet is 10 to 15 percent of calories. Research indicates that lowering fat intake to 10 percent of calories does not increase weight loss or improve cholesterol levels any more than having fat at 15 percent. A diet that contains 15 percent fat is easier to prepare and easier to maintain over the long run—you're more likely to adopt such a diet as a lifestyle change and not consider it a "diet."

Now that people have been eating low-fat diets for a number of years, scientists are able to study the effects of such diets. They're finding that if people eat less than 10 percent of calories from fat for very long, they actually experience adverse effects:

- Higher blood cholesterol levels
- Higher blood triglyceride levels
- Higher blood sugar levels
- Higher insulin levels

These four factors set the stage for heart disease. People who thought that if cutting some fat from the diet was good, then cutting even more was better, actually ended up in poorer health. The body likes moderation in all things, and this apparently includes fat. So in your eagerness to drop the pounds, don't drop all of the dietary fat.

Figuring out how much fat is in a food when it has a label is easy—that will be explained shortly—but for foods that you make or that don't have labels on them, think about what the typical ingredients are. For instance, muffins are nothing short of small cakes. They're packed with fat and sugar, even though they don't look like it. Anything that has oil, butter, cheese, cream, or other fats added to it are suspect.

Watch the Fat

Not only is it necessary to maintain some fat in the diet, but the type of fat you eat is important, too. Here's the lowdown:

Saturated Fats—These fats are called "saturated" because chemically speaking, all of their bonds are saturated with hydrogen. But what's important to remember is that saturated fat is one of the least healthful of the fats. Saturated fat causes the blood's cholesterol level to rise, which can cause clogs in important arteries. Saturated fat is found in animal foods such as meat and dairy products, as well as in vegetable

FERRETING OUT FAT

Simple ways to cut the fat:

- Make the move to skim milk. If you can't do it "cold turkey," switch first to two percent, then one percent, then skim.

- Build your meals around whole grains, beans, and vegetables. Include a variety of grains and plant foods, like barley, bulgur, couscous, oats, maybe even getting adventurous with millet, quinoa, and teff.

- Experiment with low-fat and fat-free foods on the market. Some work; some don't. In general, low-fat (one or two grams of fat per serving) cookies and crackers fare better than fat-free cookies and crackers. The fat-free cheeses are more of a gamble; some lose their ability to melt. Fat-free dressings and condiments are a good bet because you don't eat them solo, so you're less likely to miss the fat.

- Substitute plain, nonfat yogurt for sour cream.

- Use evaporated skim milk instead of cream in recipes.

- Switch to a "diet" or "light" margarine for everyday uses. But don't substitute them in baked goods because you'll be disappointed with the final product.

- Stick to whole-grain breads for everyday uses. For variety, supplement that with bagels, English muffins, French and Italian bread, pita bread, and corn tortillas.

- Use the "napkin test" on baked goods: Lay the item on a napkin; if you see a grease stain, the item is loaded with fat. Croissants are notoriously high in fat, as are most muffins, biscuits, scones, doughnuts, and pastries.

oils that make you think of warm places, such as coconut and palm kernel oil. Steer clear of saturated fats as much as possible. They should make up no more than a third of the total fats you eat.

Monounsaturated Fats—*Mono* means one, and these fats have one place in their structure where there's a double bond without hydrogen. What this means to you is that it's healthier. In fact, monounsaturated fats are considered to be the most healthful of the fats. They do not cause a rise in cholesterol levels the way saturated fats do; in fact, they help to lower the low-density lipoprotein (LDL), or "bad," cholesterol level in your blood. Monounsaturated fats are predominant in olive oil and canola oil.

Polyunsaturated Fats—*Poly* means many, and polyunsaturated fats have many double bonds where there is no hydrogen. However, they are only a moderately healthy fat. It's true that they do not cause a rise in cholesterol like saturated fat does, but there are other problems. Polyunsaturated fats' double bonds are susceptible to attack by free radicals, which can destroy some of their bonds and allow rancidity to set in. Free radicals damage not only the polyunsaturated fat does, but also cells. High intakes of this type of fat have been associated with an increased rate of cancer. Additionally, these fats tend to lower your high-density lipoprotein (HDL), or "good," cholesterol levels even though they also lower your "bad" LDL cholesterol levels. Polyunsaturated fats are the main type of fat in most vegetable oils, such as safflower, soybean, and corn oils. Use this type of fat sparingly.

Hydrogenated Fats—These fats are polyunsaturated fats that have had hydrogen forced onto the double bonds, making

YOUR DAILY FAT BUDGET

Here's a chart that shows what your daily fat budget would be if you maintained 15 percent of calories from fat.

Average calorie intake	Daily Fat Budget (for 15% fat), in grams
1,000	17
1,200	20
1,400	23
1,600 (Many women, most older adults)	27
1,800	30
2,000	33
2,200 (Active women, teen girls, most men)	37
2,400	40
2,600	43
2,800 (Teen boys, active men)	47

them a saturated fat. And the body isn't fooled; it treats them just like saturated fat, causing cholesterol levels to rise. Research shows that hydrogenated fats—sometimes called *trans* fats, short for *trans* fatty acids—disrupt cell membranes and cause cellular damage. These fats are linked to cancer and decreased immune function. Be diligent about limiting the amount of hydrogenated fats you eat. Unfortunately, this can be rather difficult, since food manufacturers put it in most processed and packaged products.

Essential Fats—These are the essential fatty acids your body cannot make. These fats promote a favorable cholesterol ratio in your blood. (You're aiming for HDL cholesterol levels to be more than 35 mg/dL, LDL cholesterol levels to be less than 130 mg/dL, and total cholesterol levels to be less than 200 mg/dL). In addition, the prostaglandins that essential fats prompt the body to make will also keep blood pressure in line, keep the blood from clotting too easily, and keep a lid on inflammation. The omega-3 essential fatty acids are abundant in fish, especially fatty fish such as salmon, tuna, albacore, herring, sardines, mackerel, bluefish, and Atlantic halibut. The omega-6 fatty acids are found in most vegetable oils, particularly safflower, corn, and sunflower oils.

Despite the "good" and "bad" fats, remember: All fats carry nine calories per gram and count in your total fat intake. Even if all your daily fat intake comes from monounsaturated fat, you still need to limit it to 15 percent of calories. Fat—even the beneficial kind—adds up in terms of calories.

SORTING IT OUT WITH LABELS

When comparing products to decide which will fit into your low-fat, high-carbohydrate eating plan, the Nutrition Facts portion of the label will come in handy.

First, look at the serving size. Is this about how much you eat at one time? If not, you'll need to adjust the numbers on the label accordingly. For instance, if the serving size is one-half cup but you normally eat about one cup at a time, then you'll need to double all the numbers on the label.

Here are some tips on what to look for on food labels:

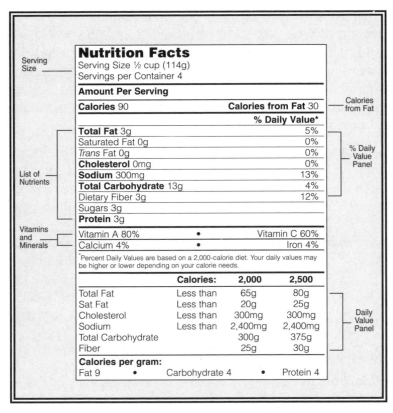

Serving Size →	**Nutrition Facts**	

Nutrition Facts
Serving Size ½ cup (114g)
Servings per Container 4

Amount Per Serving

Calories 90	**Calories from Fat** 30

	% Daily Value*
Total Fat 3g	5%
Saturated Fat 0g	0%
Trans Fat 0g	0%
Cholesterol 0mg	0%
Sodium 300mg	13%
Total Carbohydrate 13g	4%
Dietary Fiber 3g	12%
Sugars 3g	
Protein 3g	

Vitamin A 80%	•	Vitamin C 60%
Calcium 4%	•	Iron 4%

*Percent Daily Values are based on a 2,000-calorie diet. Your daily values may be higher or lower depending on your calorie needs.

	Calories:	2,000	2,500
Total Fat	Less than	65g	80g
Sat Fat	Less than	20g	25g
Cholesterol	Less than	300mg	300mg
Sodium	Less than	2,400mg	2,400mg
Total Carbohydrate		300g	375g
Fiber		25g	30g

Calories per gram:
Fat 9 • Carbohydrate 4 • Protein 4

(Labels: Serving Size, List of Nutrients, Vitamins and Minerals, Calories from Fat, % Daily Value Panel, Daily Value Panel)

Total Fat tells you how many grams of fat are in one serving. The percentage to the right, called the *% Daily Value*, tells you how much of your daily fat budget is used up by one serving of the food, if you typically eat 2,000 calories and aim to get 30 percent of your calories from fat. You, however, are on a slightly different track because you're aiming for about 15 percent of calories from fat and your calorie intake may be considerably lower than 2,000. It's easiest just to use the grams of total fat and keep them tallied throughout the day.

In addition to total fat, the labels are required to list the amount of saturated fat in a product. Remember to choose foods that are low in saturated fat, since this is not a healthy type of fat. Some labels voluntarily list amounts of monounsaturated and polyunsaturated fats too, and you can use this information to choose products that are higher in monounsaturated fats and lower in polyunsaturated fats.

And, finally, the government recently ruled that, no later than January 2006, each food label must list the amount of *trans* fat in the product. *Trans* fat, which is fat that has been hydrogenated, is similar to saturated fat and cholesterol in its neg-

Label Lingo

Finally, manufacturers are being held accountable for those claims they make on food labels. Here is what they have to mean:

Low calorie—40 calories or less per serving

Light or Lite—⅓ fewer calories or 50% less fat than the regular version

Fat free—less than 0.5 gram of fat per serving

Low fat—3 grams or less of fat per serving

Low cholesterol—20 milligrams or less per serving

Lean—fewer than 10 grams total fat, 4 grams saturated fat, *and* 95 milligrams cholesterol per serving

Extra lean—fewer than 5 grams total fat, 2 grams saturated fat, *and* 95 milligrams cholesterol per serving

ative effects on heart health. So you can use all of this fat information on food labels to choose foods that are not only lower in fat but that provide healthier types of fat.

If you need to watch your salt or sodium intake, pay attention to that portion of the label, too. Reduced-fat foods often have more salt added to them to make up for the flavor that the fat contributed.

Next, check out the amount of fiber in the food. Dietary fiber is listed beneath *Total Carbohydrates*. Remember all the benefits of fiber, and choose foods that have as much as possible. For example, when choosing a loaf of bread, select one that offers two or more grams of fiber per slice, rather than one that offers only one or none.

Also beneath the *Total Carbohydrates* section you'll find sugars. If the product does not contain fruit or dairy products, then you can be assured that the amount listed comes from added sugars. Whether it's white table sugar—known as sucrose—or corn syrup or honey, they all provide calories and few nutrients. Keep your total added sugar intake below 50 grams per day. Products containing milk and primarily fruit don't count, because the natural sugars in these items are combined with any added sugars that might be present. It's impossible to know from labels on these foods how much sugar is added and how much occurs naturally.

PICK YOUR PROTEIN

Yes, even complex carbohydrates can provide all the protein you need. It's just a matter of know-how when it comes to combining them. Cultures all around the world have done this well for thousands of years. Meat was not always available and, in more modern times, may not be affordable. Yet people are strong, healthy, and robust, consuming little or no meat.

Complex carbohydrates contain not only starches, but substances called amino acids, which are the building blocks of protein. There are many amino acids, but the body is unable to make eight or nine of them, depending on your stage of life. So these particular amino acids are considered essential and must be obtained from food.

The problem is that most foods contain an abundance of certain essential amino acids while they lack other essential ones. So foods must be combined or eaten together in order to provide the body with all the essential amino acids in good proportions. Don't despair, though; it's much easier than it sounds.

By combining these foods it's usually very easy—and delicious—to get the amino acids your body needs. Even if you don't combine the appropriate foods within one meal, it's OK to combine them within the same day or even over a period of a couple days. Amino acids float throughout your system all the time, and they'll wait a day or two to hitch up with just the right one they need.

Most Americans eat twice as much protein as they need, so don't be concerned about getting enough. As long as you include beans, grains, and dairy foods, you'll be set. Even athletes don't need huge amounts of protein. Muscle strength and endurance is based on repeated exercise and consumption of complex carbohydrates. Protein merely builds the matrix that the body fills with carbohydrates to make muscles grow.

AMINO ACID ARITHMETIC

Combine these foods to make complete proteins your body can use:

Legumes with Grains

> Legumes include all dry beans, peanuts, split peas, and lentils. Examples of this combination are: pinto beans with corn tortillas, black beans with rice, peanut butter on bread, tofu (made from soybeans) with rice, lentil or split pea soup with wheat or rye bread, black-eyed peas with cornbread.

Grains with Dairy

> For instance, cereal and skim milk, toast with nonfat yogurt, sandwich and skim milk.

Legumes with Seeds and Nuts

> Top a bean dish with a sprinkle of toasted almonds or sesame seeds, make humus with garbanzo beans and sesame seeds, or mix up a tofu and cashew stir-fry to serve over rice.

Too much protein can actually be detrimental, as discussed earlier. Protein, especially from animal products, can tax the kidneys, make you dehydrated, and even leach calcium from your bones. Animal proteins are also often accompanied by quite a bit of fat and cholesterol, things you're trying to cut down on. Meeting your protein needs with mostly complex carbohydrates is the healthy and weight-dropping way to go.

As you probably know, nuts are high in fat, but mostly monounsaturated fat, the healthy kind. Still, you don't want to overdo it. Nuts are rich in protein and minerals, so it's a good idea to occasionally include small amounts. For example, toast chopped nuts in a dry skillet until they're fragrant and golden brown, then sprinkle over rice. Limit your intake of nuts to two tablespoons per day.

Fish is another excellent protein source that goes well with many complex carbohydrates. Are you one of those people who say, "I don't like fish"? Perhaps it would help if you tried a very mild variety, such as cod. Find a cookbook on fish at your public library or bookstore and fix fish in ways you have never tried before. Who could resist baked cod encrusted with toasted bread crumbs and served with lemon and dill? It's important to include fish because of the heart-healthy omega-3 fatty acids they contain. In fact, the fattier the fish, the more of these precious fats you'll get. So this is one arena in which it's alright to eat moderate amounts of a high-fat food—as long as the fat is naturally in the fish and not added fat. Eat fish in 3- to 4-ounce serving sizes, which is about the size of a deck of cards, several times per week.

The omega-3 fatty acids in fish can actually benefit your weight-loss plan because they help the body metabolize fat well—so that too much fat doesn't end up in your bloodstream on its way to be deposited into fat cells.

YOU CAN STILL ENJOY EATING OUT

It's fun to eat out, and any eating plan that doesn't make room for you to do so is not one you're likely to stick with for long. By studying the menu and asking your server a few questions, you can get an enjoyable meal that fits into your eating regime.

First, scan the menu for vegetarian or fish entrées. The vegetarian entrée will undoubtedly be rich in complex carbohydrates, but beware of what might be added to it. Identify added ingredients (see chart below) such as a cream sauce, as in fettuccine Alfredo. If available, choose a red sauce, which will be based on tomatoes rather than on cream or butter.

Be aware, too, of words used to describe how the item is prepared. Is it fried or baked? Sautéed or steamed? Choose preparation methods that use little or no fat. Ask your server questions if it's not clear on the menu, or if it doesn't say. Some people are too shy to ask, but keep in mind that the server is there to serve you—you're paying for their time as well as the food so you might as well make use of their knowledge.

Make special requests when eating out. For instance, ask for salad dressing on the side, or if you've ordered anything from pancakes to a baked potato, ask for the butter and other top-

BE A MENU SLEUTH

Be on the lookout for ten telltale words that, when translated, loosely mean "fat":

Alfredo	Creamy
Batter-dipped	Crispy
Béarnaise	Stuffed
Béchamel	Supreme
Breaded	Tempura

pings on the side. Anytime you can, get the sauce or toppings served separately so that you can control how much you eat of them. Dipping your fork first into the salad dressing then forking a bit of lettuce will still give you plenty of flavor with hardly any fat. If you find it difficult to make special requests, practice at home before going out.

Planning ahead is instrumental in eating out, too, whether you're going to a restaurant, a banquet, or a friend's house. Think about what's likely to be served, and plan the things you'll look for to eat. Advance planning is a remarkable way to prevent temptation and overeating. For example, you might plan to eat tossed salad if you expect to splurge on dessert. It's often a good idea to eat a low-calorie snack beforehand to dull your appetite. Also plan what you'll say to politely decline food that doesn't fit into your eating pattern, especially if it's friends or relatives who will be offering.

Fast food can occasionally fit into your complex carbohydrate plan, too. Just be picky about your choices. When given the chance, choose a fast food restaurant that has reasonable options. For instance, at some Mexican fast food places, there are bean and rice burritos or wraps available—just beware of sauces. Fast food fish places typically offer a baked or grilled version in addition to breaded and fried. Quick teriyaki places are ideal, as you can get heaps of rice and steamed vegetables instantly. At a hamburger restaurant, it gets a little tougher— sometimes a salad and bread are the best you can find.

Whichever fast food restaurant you choose, be sure to ask for a nutrition brochure. Most chains have them behind the counter. The brochure will tell you not only which items are full of carbohydrates, but also the fat and calorie content of each menu item so that you can make an informed choice. Collect the brochures from the fast food restaurants you typically go to, look them over, and plan your order options at each of them so you'll be ready when the time comes.

ACTIVITY: THE FINAL INGREDIENT

You've heard it before. You know it's true. But now there are more reasons than ever to get moving!

For starters, did you know that for several hours after physical activity your metabolic rate stays elevated? That's right. If you take a brisk walk or go cycling while your spouse stays home, then come back and you both watch TV, you'll be burning more calories than your spouse for several hours, just because you exercised. Activity raises your metabolic rate while you're doing it, plus it takes one to three hours for it to return to previous levels.

Another bonus: Whenever you're active, you're building lean muscle tissue. Even if you're just walking around the block a few times, you're toning your muscles more than if you were reading a book. The more muscle you have, the higher your metabolic rate will be. If you're getting more muscular and your spouse is flabby, and you're both sitting around playing cards, you're going to be burning more calories than your spouse is, automatically, just because you have more muscle tissue.

Whenever you can raise your metabolic rate, you're promoting weight loss. The rate at which you burn calories while at rest is one of the biggest burners of calories all day long. So if you can pump it up to be burning more even when you're not active, you'll shed pounds more easily.

Assuming your goal is to lose weight, it's important to do aerobic exercise as well as strength-training exercises. Aerobic activity, such as brisk walking, cycling, jogging, swimming, and so forth, helps you lose fat tissue. During the first 20 minutes of aerobic activity, your body burns mostly stored carbohydrates and just a little bit of fat. But at the 20-minute mark, something wondrous happens. Your body shifts gears and begins to burn more fat. Visualize it this way: at the 20-minute mark, an alarm goes off and your control center commands fat cells to open up and release their load. And they do! You start burning mostly fat after 20 minutes of exercise. So the best way to get rid of unwanted fat is to keep moving for more than 20 minutes to take full benefit of your body's fat-burning command mechanism.

How do you know if you're exercising aerobically? Aerobic exercise is when the heart and lungs can still keep up with the oxygen demands of the muscles. If you're breathing rate is increased but you're still able to talk while you're exercising—without too much huffing and puffing—you're in an aerobic state. If you overdo it and go beyond this point, you push your body into anaerobic metabolism, and you don't burn any fat at all. So aim for a more moderate pace, and keep talking. Be sure to check with your doctor before undertaking any new exercise regime.

The other type of activity that will make it easier for you to drop unwanted pounds is to do strength training. You can even do this in front of the TV! Strength training builds and tones muscles. And remember, the more muscle tissue you have, the more calories you'll burn even when resting because of the boost it gives to your metabolism.

HOW MANY CALORIES DO YOU BURN?

Weight (in pounds)....100	130	150	170	190	210
	Calories Burned Per Hour*				
Basketball 414	486	564	636	714	786
Card playing..................78	90	102	114	132	144
Cycling (9.4 mph)........300	354	408	462	516	570
Eating............................72	84	96	108	120	132
Fishing, active.............186	222	252	288	318	354
Running (11.5 minutes per mile) 408	480	552	630	702	774
Swimming, slow crawl stroke.....384	456	522	594	660	732
Tennis..........................330	384	444	504	564	624
Walking, normal pace 240	282	324	372	414	456

*These are estimates; the actual number of calories you burn during these activities may vary.

Start with one-pound weights and your favorite show. Purchase weights or use plastic one-gallon milk or water jugs partially filled with water or sand. Stand in front of the TV and lift the weights out to the side, over your head, in front of you—any way that's comfortable. (Stop if you have pain.) Start out with three sets of 12 to 15 repetitions. When you can do those easily, increase the weights slightly. Continue until you build up to three- or five-pound weights for each hand. Increased repetitions will tone, whereas increased weight will build muscle. Both are important.

To develop your leg muscles, get ankle weights or use resealable plastic bags each filled with a pound of rice or sand. Strap on the ankle weights or use rubber bands to attach the weighted plastic bags. Do sitting and standing leg lifts, 12 to 15 repetitions, three times. Again, these can be done painlessly as you concentrate on your favorite TV show. Increase the weights as you're able, building up over the course of several weeks or months.

Alternate aerobic and strength-training exercises on an every-other-day basis. Muscles need a day in between workouts to recuperate; so alternating activities is ideal.

GET GOING!

Now that you know the basics, it's time to look over the food profiles and begin to plan your new eating habits. Clean out your cupboards, give away foods you no longer want, and make a list of all the delicious new foods you can stock up on. Eat simply, stay active, and enjoy!

AMARANTH

This ancient grain of the Aztecs has been recently rediscovered by Westerners, although you'll probably need to visit a health-food store or check a mail-order catalog to find it. Technically, it's not a grain; it's the fruit of a plant. And that's the reason it contains a more complete protein, and more of it, than other traditional grains. It has a distinctive sweet but peppery taste—one that many people prefer combined with other grains, for a more mellow flavor.

HEALTH BENEFITS

Even when just a little is included in a recipe, the benefit is worth it. For anyone cutting down on meat, amaranth offers a bonanza of near-complete protein. It's not missing the amino acid lysine, as many grains are. It is also much richer in iron, magnesium, and calcium than most grains, so it can help keep anemia and osteoporosis at bay. It excels as a source of fiber, mostly insoluble, which is of help in reducing the risk of a variety of diseases, including certain cancers and digestive-tract conditions.

SELECTION AND STORAGE

Amaranth is a tiny, yellow grain. It can be bought as a whole grain ("pearled" amaranth), as a flour, or as rolled flakes. It's also found as an ingredient in cereals and crackers. Expect to pay more for it; amaranth is not widely grown and is difficult to harvest, so it is more expensive than other grains. But, remember, you get a lot of nutritional bang for your buck.

Keep amaranth in a tightly closed container to prevent insect infestation. And store in a cool, dry location to prevent the fat in it from turning rancid.

Preparation and Serving Tips

This versatile grain can be cooked in liquids and eaten as a porridge or pilaf. It can even be popped like corn. But because of its strong flavor, you may like it best combined with other grains. For baking, amaranth must be combined with another flour, such as wheat, because it contains no gluten by itself.

To cook: Cook one cup of grains in three cups of water (yield: three cups). Bring to a boil, then simmer for 25 minutes. The final consistency will be thick, like porridge. If you want to cook it with another grain, such as oatmeal or rice, just substitute amaranth for about a quarter of the other grain, then cook as you would for that grain.

To pop: Stir a tablespoon at a time over high heat, in an ungreased skillet, until the grain pops, like corn. This can be used as a breading for fish or chicken or to top salads and soups.

AMARANTH
Serving Size: ¼ cup dry, uncooked

Calories	183	Calcium	75 mg
Protein	7.1 g	Copper	0.4 mg
Carbohydrate	32.4 g	Iron	3.71 mg
Fat	3.2 g	Magnesium	130 mg
Saturated	0.8 g	Phosphorus	223 mg
Cholesterol	0 mg	Potassium	179.5 mg
Dietary Fiber	5.1 g	Zinc	1.6 mg
Sodium	10.5 mg		

APPLES

Chances are, you've only tasted a few of the many varieties of apples because supermarkets offer a small selection that typically includes Cortland, Granny Smith, McIntosh, and the most popular—Red Delicious. Regardless of the type, apples are a perfect addition to your fat-fighting diet since they provide ample amounts of fiber. Enjoying a fiber-packed apple, especially before a meal, is a good way to curb your appetite. It's also a great low-fat snack when you're on the run.

HEALTH BENEFITS

Even though it's not bursting with nutrients like some of the other fruits, an apple a day may do more than keep the doctor away. For starters, apples are a good source of vitamin C, an antioxidant, and research has shown that antioxidants may help prevent the formation of some cancers. They have heart-healthy effects, too—apples are loaded with pectin, which may keep blood cholesterol levels in check. Plus, when it dissolves in water, soluble fiber creates a gummy, gel-like substance that binds bile acids and draws cholesterol out of the bloodstream. Soluble fiber's stickiness also ties up carbohydrates, keeping blood sugar levels on an even keel. And apples may contribute to a healthy smile and fresh breath by stimulating your gums and promoting saliva production.

SELECTION AND STORAGE

A few varieties, like Cortland, Jonathan, and Winesap, are all-purpose apples. But in general, choose apples for their intended purpose. For baking, try Golden Delicious, Rome

— APPLES

Beauty, Cortland, Northern Spy, or Rhode Island Greening; they deliver flavor and keep their shape when cooked. For just plain eating, you can't beat tart Macouns or award-winning Empires.

If possible, buy apples from an orchard. Apples prefer humid air, so the crisper drawer of the refrigerator is the best place to store them. Some varieties will keep until spring, though most get mealy in a month or two. Golden Delicious must be enjoyed right away before their skins shrivel.

PREPARATION AND SERVING TIPS

Always wash and scrub your apples. Though Alar, the infamous pesticide, is no longer used by apple growers, supermarket apples are often waxed, which seals in pesticide residues that may be on the skins. Peeling apples will remove the film but also a lot of the fiber. All apples will brown when cut, but the rate varies among varieties. To prevent browning, sprinkle a little lemon juice on cut surfaces.

APPLE, FRESH
Serving Size: 1 small

Calories....................81	Protein ....<1 g
Fat.............................1 g	Dietary Fiber...............3 g
Saturated Fat.......<1 g	Sodium.......................1 mg
Cholesterol.................0 mg	Vitamin C ....8 mg
Carbohydrate ....21 g	

APRICOTS

Despite their size, fresh apricots are well-suited for low-fat diets because they are particularly rich in fiber, especially insoluble, which absorbs water and helps contribute to a feeling of fullness. But their fragrant aroma alone makes fresh apricots a dieter's delight.

HEALTH BENEFITS

Apricots are also abundant in good-for-your-heart soluble fiber, which dissolves in water to form gels that bind with bile acids, forcing your body to draw cholesterol from the bloodstream to make more bile acids. But the real heart-healthy news about apricots is that they are brimming with beta-carotene—an important antioxidant that's a member of the vitamin A family. Researchers have linked beta-carotene–rich foods to the prevention of certain cancers (especially lung), cataracts, and heart disease.

Since this fruit's season is short and sweet, canned and dried apricots offer a delicious alternative to fresh. Canned apricots, unfortunately, are not nutritionally equivalent to the fresh variety; sugar is often added during the canning process, and the high heat used in the process cuts the amount of beta-carotene and vitamin C in half.

The drying process concentrates the carbohydrates, so a single serving contains a hefty amount of calories. In fact, a half-cup serving of dried apricots yields three times the calories of a single serving of fresh. So read the labels and pay attention to serving sizes to make sure your portions don't play a role in a calorie overload.

APRICOTS, FRESH
Serving Size: 3 medium

Calories	51	Dietary Fiber	3 g
Fat	1 g	Sodium	1 mg
Saturated Fat	0 g	Vitamin A	2,769 IU
Cholesterol	0 mg	Vitamin C	11 mg
Carbohydrate	12 g	Potassium	313 mg
Protein	2 g		

SELECTION AND STORAGE

Apricots are delicate and must be handled with care. One of the easiest ways to preserve these fragile gems is for growers to pick them before they are ripe. So you'll need to ripen the fruit for a day or two at room temperature before you can enjoy them. But don't pile them up or the pressure will cause them to bruise as they ripen. Once they are ripe, store them in the refrigerator.

For the best flavor and nutrition, look for plump, golden-orange apricots that are fairly firm or yield slightly to thumb pressure. Avoid those that are tinged with green or have a pale yellow color; they were picked too soon.

PREPARATION AND SERVING TIPS

Be gentle when washing fresh apricots or they'll bruise. To reap the fat-fighting benefits of apricots, it's best to eat them skins and all. But if you would rather peel them, here's an easy way to get the job done fast: Dip the apricot in boiling water for 30 seconds, then immediately peel with a sharp knife under cold running water.

ARTICHOKES

Fibrous artichokes are a dieter's delight—low in fat and loaded with fiber. Yet many would-be artichoke lovers shy away from this delicate, buttery-flavored vegetable since they don't know how to handle it. Actually, artichokes require little prep work; the time-consuming step is the process of eating—that's why this odd vegetable should be included in your low-fat diet. Because it's labor-intensive to consume, you are forced to eat at a leisurely pace, giving your stomach time to tell your brain it's full, which may prevent you from overeating.

HEALTH BENEFITS

Artichokes' high fiber content is also a bonus for your digestive tract. Insoluble fiber is nature's laxative, absorbing water and creating bulk to move things along. Artichokes are also a super source of folic acid, which is especially important for women during their childbearing years, as this vitamin helps prevent neural-tube birth defects. New research has also linked long-term deficiencies of folic acid to an increased risk of developing heart disease.

SELECTION AND STORAGE

Green globe artichokes are grown in the United States. Baby artichokes come from a side thistle of the plant; artichoke hearts are the meaty base. A Jerusalem artichoke is not an artichoke at all; it's an unrelated root vegetable.

Look for heavy artichokes with a soft green color and tightly packed, closed leaves. Bronzed or frosted leaf tips signal delicate flavor. Avoid moldy or wilted leaves.

ARTICHOKE, FRESH, COOKED
Serving Size: 1 medium

Calories	53	Sodium	79 mg
Fat	<1 g	Vitamin C	9 mg
Saturated Fat	0 g	Folic Acid	53 mcg
Cholesterol	0 mg	Iron	2 mg
Carbohydrate	12 g	Magnesium	47 mg
Protein	3 g	Manganese	<1 mg
Dietary Fiber	6 g	Potassium	316 mg

Store artichokes in a plastic bag in the refrigerator; add a few drops of water to prevent them from drying out. (Do not wash artichokes before storing them.) Although best if used within a few days, they'll keep for a week or two if stored properly and handled gently.

PREPARATION AND SERVING TIPS

Wash artichokes under running water. Pull off outer, lower petals and trim the sharp tips off of the outer leaves. Boil, standing upright in the saucepan, for 20 to 40 minutes, or steam for 25 to 40 minutes or until a center petal pulls out easily.

Artichokes are versatile; they can be served hot, at room temperature, or cold. Though they're best served as appetizers, they are well suited for a variety of uses including dips and sauces. Or stick to plain lemon juice. Butter, of course, is a no-no for those who want less flab and more muscle.

ASPARAGUS

This vegetable has garnered a reputation for being elitist, probably because it's rather expensive when bought out of season. But if you're like many people, you may swear it's worth its weight in gold. Gourmet or not, you can't beat the nutrition you get for what asparagus "costs" calorie-wise. At less than four calories a spear, you can't go wrong unless you unwisely top it with Hollandaise sauce. Asparagus not only has few calories, but it also has major flavor, which is often missing in many of the new low-fat and fat-free products in the supermarkets. Most people like to savor their spears, a practice that extends the dining experience and so may prevent you from overindulging in other foods.

HEALTH BENEFITS

Asparagus is ideal for young women; it's a winner when it comes to folic acid—a vitamin that helps prevent neural-tube birth defects. Two major antioxidants—beta-carotene and vitamin C—are also abundant in asparagus. By neutralizing damaging particles in our bodies like smog and cigarette smoke, antioxidants are thought to be major contenders in the fight against heart disease, cancer, and cataracts.

SELECTION AND STORAGE

Spotting the first asparagus in stores is a sign of early spring. Look for a bright green color; stalks that are smooth, firm, straight, and round, not flat; and tips that are compact, closed, pointed, and purplish in color. Thick stalks are fine, but choose stalks of similar size so they'll cook at the same rate.

Asparagus, Fresh, Cooked
Serving Size: 4 spears

Calories....................15	Dietary Fiber ....1 g
Fat...........................<1 g	Sodium.......................3 mg
Saturated Fat.........0 g	Vitamin A................498 IU
Cholesterol.................0 mg	Vitamin C ....16 mg
Carbohydrate ....3 g	Folic Acid ....59 mcg
Protein.......................2 g	Potassium ....186 mg

Keep asparagus cold or the stalks will deteriorate, losing flavor and vitamin C. Wrapped loosely in a plastic bag, the stalks will keep for almost a week. To enjoy asparagus year-round, blanch the spears the day you buy them, wrap them tightly in foil, and freeze for up to 12 months.

PREPARATION AND SERVING TIPS

Snap off the whitish stem ends. Add these to soup stock instead of just tossing them out. Boil, steam, or microwave asparagus, but avoid overcooking it. When cooked correctly, the spears should be crisp-tender and bright green. Overcooked spears turn mushy and a drab olive green. Simmer for three to five minutes only. For more even cooking, stand stalks upright in boiling water, with the tips sticking out of the water, for five to ten minutes. This way, the tips steam as the stalks cook. Microwaving takes two to three minutes in a dish with a quarter-cup water. You can serve asparagus hot, warm, or cold. For a change of pace, try adding cut-up asparagus to your next stir-fry or pasta dish.

BANANAS

Bananas come in their own perfect package, so there's no mess, no fuss—they're the perfect take-along snack. No wonder they're one of the most popular fruits in the United States. Admittedly higher in calories than most other fruits, their calories are nearly fat-free calories.

HEALTH BENEFITS

Bananas are loaded with potassium, and researchers now believe that adding potassium may play a stronger role in the control of high blood pressure than restricting salt. Magnesium is also abundant; many researchers think this mineral helps keep blood pressure levels in check, too.

Generally, fruit is a poor source of vitamin B_6, but bananas are the exception; a single serving has more than 30 percent of the RDA. Vitamin B_6 helps to keep your immune system performing at its peak, and recent studies have found that, like a deficiency of folic acid, a long-term deficiency of B_6 may increase your risk of heart disease.

SELECTION AND STORAGE

There are different types of bananas, but Cavendish, the yellow bananas, are the most familiar. To appeal to a variety of cultures, supermarkets are now expanding their selections to include red bananas and plantains, those seemingly underripe bananas that never lose their mossy green color.

Most bananas ripen after picking, and as they do, the starch in them turns to sugar. So the riper they are, the sweeter they

BANANA, YELLOW
Serving Size: 1 (8½-inch) banana

Calories	105	Sodium	1 mg
Fat	1 g	Vitamin C	10 mg
Saturated Fat	<1 g	Vitamin B_6	1 mg
Cholesterol	0 mg	Magnesium	33 mg
Carbohydrate	27 g	Manganese	<1 mg
Protein	1 g	Potassium	451 mg
Dietary Fiber	2 g		

are. Look for plump, firm bananas with no bruises or split skins. Brown spots are a sign of ripening. If your banana skins are tinged with green, allow them to ripen at room temperature (don't refrigerate unripe bananas; they'll never ripen); refrigerate them once they are ripe to stop the process. They'll turn an unsightly, but harmless, black color.

PREPARATION AND SERVING TIPS

Yellow bananas are great on their own, but when mashed, they make a great low-fat, nutrient-packed spread for toasted bagels. Sprinkle lemon juice on banana slices to keep them from darkening. To salvage bananas that are too ripe, combine them in a blender with orange juice and skim milk for a healthful "smoothie"—a great take-along treat for dashboard dining. For the kids, try frozen banana pops: Peel and cut a banana in half; insert a craft stick into each half. Dip the bananas into orange juice, roll them in wheat germ, and freeze them until they are firm.

BARLEY

When baked in casseroles, stuffed into vegetables, or served in place of rice, this flavorful, fiber-packed, Middle Eastern grain curbs your appetite for higher-fat fare—the bulking ability of fiber fills you up and reduces the likelihood that you'll overindulge in fat and calories.

HEALTH BENEFITS

You may have heard about oat bran and its cholesterol-lowering ability; new research suggests that barley may have a similar effect on cholesterol, too. Barley contains the same cholesterol-fighting soluble fiber, beta-glucan, found in oat bran and dry beans. Farmers are jumping on the bandwagon and are growing varieties—such as hulless and waxy barley—that are super-high in beta-glucan. The soluble fiber pectin fights cholesterol, too.

Barley is rich in insoluble fiber as well; the whole, hulled form contains more than whole wheat. As insoluble fiber absorbs water, it adds bulk and speeds intestinal contents through your body, which may reduce your risk of developing colorectal cancers since contact between harmful substances and your intestinal wall is limited. And there's another bonus—insoluble fiber may help keep digestive disorders, like constipation and hemorrhoid flare-ups, at bay.

SELECTION AND STORAGE

Whole, hulled barley—brown, unpearled—is the most nutritious. It has twice the fiber and more than twice the vitamins and minerals of pearled. It's available in health-food stores.

Scotch barley, or pot barley, is refined less than the pearled type, so part of the bran's goodness remains.

Pearled barley is the easiest variety to find. While nutritionally inferior to the other two types, it boasts decent fiber and iron, and it is certainly not devoid of nutrients.

Store pearled and Scotch barley in airtight containers in a cool, dark location for up to one year; nine months for all other varieties.

PREPARATION AND SERVING TIPS

To cook: Add one cup of pearled barley to three cups of boiling water (or one cup of whole barley to four cups of boiling water). Simmer, covered, for 45 to 55 minutes (1 hour to 1 hour 40 minutes for whole barley).

As barley cooks, the starch in it swells and absorbs water, making it soft and bulky. This makes it the perfect thickener for soups, stews, and traditional Scotch broth soup. Barley can be successfully substituted for rice in almost any recipe. It has more flavor than white rice though it isn't as strong as brown rice—the perfect compromise.

BARLEY, PEARLED, COOKED
Serving Size: ½ cup

Calories...................97	Dietary Fiber..............4 g
Fat............................<1 g	Sodium.......................2 mg
Saturated Fat.......<1 g	Niacin........................2 mg
Cholesterol................ 0 mg	Iron............................1 mg
Carbohydrate ....22 g	Manganese ....<1 mg
Protein.......................2 g	

Beans & Peas, Dry

If you had to pick one food to be stuck on a desert island with, it would have to be beans. They'd provide you with almost complete nutrition and you wouldn't have to worry about offending anyone. Yes, beans can be gassy, but there are ways around that. So don't let their "explosive" nature scare you away from some of the best fat-fighting nutrition around.

When your diet's based on beans and other complex carbohydrates, you're more likely to follow a low-fat, high-fiber diet. Complementing beans with other low-fat types of protein, like rice, makes them a great substitute for high-fat protein sources like meats. Beans are also filling enough to stave off hunger. The low-fat, high-fiber nature of a bean-centered diet means that chances are good that you'll lose weight eating this way.

Health Benefits

Not only are beans low in fat and high in quality protein, but they also have the added bonus of soluble fiber's disease-preventing qualities. The soluble fiber in beans dissolves in water, trapping bile acids in its gummy goo. This lowers blood levels of damaging LDL cholesterol, especially if LDL cholesterol levels were high to begin with, without compromising the level of protective HDL cholesterol.

Because beans are singled out for their soluble fiber, you may not realize they also provide substantial insoluble fiber, which helps combat constipation, colon cancer, and other conditions that afflict your digestive tract. How? Insoluble fiber absorbs water, which swells the size of stool, puts pressure on the

FIBER CONTENT OF SELECTED DRY BEANS & PEAS
(grams per ½ cup serving, cooked)

Kidney beans	6.9	Great Northern beans.	5.0
Butter beans	6.9	Black-eyed peas	4.7
Navy beans	6.5	Chick-peas	
Black beans	6.1	(garbanzos)	4.3
Pinto beans	5.9	Mung beans	3.3
Broad (fava) beans	5.1	Split peas	3.1

intestines, and moves everything along faster. To help combat the gas problem—caused by indigestible carbohydrates—let your body get used to eating beans. Start slowly, eating only small amounts at first, and try to eat them when you know you'll be active afterward; it helps break up the gas.

As for vitamins and minerals, beans are a bonanza of folic acid, copper, iron, and magnesium—four nutrients that many nutrition experts agree we don't get enough of. Indeed, most dry beans and peas are rich sources of iron—ideal for people who don't eat meat.

The nutritional content of most beans is very similar to the black beans we've chosen as a representative example. (Soybeans are in a class by themselves, so are listed separately.) Exceptions? White beans have almost twice the iron of black beans, while kidney beans are somewhere in between. And fiber does vary. Most differences, however, are minor.

SELECTION AND STORAGE

Dry beans are available year-round, are inexpensive, and can be found in any well-stocked supermarket (check the ethnic food section). You may need to visit a health-food store for more exotic varieties. Packaged or loose, select beans that look clean, are not shriveled, and are uniformly sized with even color and uncracked hulls. Discard any pebbles, as well as any beans with pinholes, a sign of insect infestation. Some varieties of beans are available canned. They offer convenience but are rather mushy and very salty, although researchers have found that rinsing canned beans under cold running water for one minute eliminates up to 60 percent of the added salt.

If stored properly, dried beans last for a year or more. If packaged, keep them in their unopened bag. Once open, or if you bought them in bulk, store them in a dry, airtight glass jar in a cool, dark spot. Store cooked beans in an airtight container for up to one week in the refrigerator or freeze for up to six months.

PREPARATION AND SERVING TIPS

When cooking dry beans, it's best to plan ahead; they do not qualify as "fast" food. Before soaking or cooking, sort through the beans, discarding shriveled or discolored beans, pebbles, and debris; then rinse the beans under cold running water. It's best to soak beans overnight for six to eight hours. This softens the beans, reduces the cooking time, and removes the gas-promoting undigestible carbohydrates. But if you haven't planned far enough ahead, you can quick-soak them (although you'll end up with less-firm beans): Put the beans in water and boil for one minute, turn off the heat, and let them stand in the same water for one hour.

After soaking, discard any beans that float to the top, throw out the soaking water (which contains the gas-producing indigestible carbohydrates), and add fresh water to the pot before

Black Beans, Cooked
Serving Size: ½ cup

Calories	113	Thiamin	<1 mg
Fat	<1 g	Folic Acid	128 mcg
Saturated Fat	<1 g	Copper	<1 mg
Cholesterol	0 mg	Iron	2 g
Carbohydrate	20 g	Magnesium	60 mg
Protein	8 g	Manganese	<1 mg
Dietary Fiber	6 g	Phosphorus	120 mg
Sodium	1 mg	Potassium	306 mg

cooking. Add enough water to cover the beans by two inches. Bring to a boil, then simmer, covered, until tender—about one to three hours, depending on the bean variety. They're done when you can easily stick them with a fork.

Beans are notoriously bland-tasting, but that makes them versatile. They take on the spices of any ethnic cuisine. Many other cultures have perfected the art of combining beans with grains or seeds to provide a complete protein. For instance, try Mexican corn tortillas with beans and tomatoes, or classic Spanish rice and beans, or traditional Italian pasta e fagioli (a pasta and bean soup). You can't beat black bean soup with complementary corn bread on the side.

BEETS

Beets have only been appreciated as fat-fighting root vegetables in modern times. Before that, the beet greens were favored, most likely for their medicinal qualities, over the actual beet. Maybe back then, people were put off by the red urine and stools that sometimes appear after eating beets; some people inherit an inability to break down the red pigment in beets, so it passes right through their systems and is excreted. It's harmless enough, but you may want to lay off beets a few days before your next doctor's visit. Beets contain a wealth of fiber—half soluble and half insoluble. Both types play roles in fighting fat.

HEALTH BENEFITS

Beets are particularly rich in folic acid, calcium, and iron. Consuming adequate amounts of folic acid during the child-bearing years is a must for women; a deficiency in this critical nutrient has been linked to neural-tube birth defects. But this important vitamin is critical to life-long health for men, women, and children, because long-term deficiencies have been linked to heart disease and cervical cancer, too.

SELECTION AND STORAGE

Your best bet for beets is to choose small, firm ones that are well-rounded and uniformly sized for even cooking. The freshest beets are those with bright, crisp greens on top. The skins should be deep red, smooth, and unblemished. Thin taproots, the roots that extend from the bulb of the beets, are good indicators of tenderness.

BEETS, FRESH, COOKED
Serving Size: 2 beets

Calories	31	Dietary Fiber	3 g
Fat	<1 g	Sodium	49 mg
Saturated Fat	0 g	Folic Acid	53 mcg
Cholesterol	0 mg	Magnesium	37 mg
Carbohydrate	7 g	Manganese	<1 mg
Protein	1 g	Potassium	312 mg

Once home, cut off the greens because they suck moisture from the beets. Leave two inches of stem to prevent the beet from "bleeding" when cooked. Keep beets in a cool place; refrigerated, they'll keep for a week or two.

PREPARATION AND SERVING TIPS

Wash fresh beets gently, or broken skin will allow color and nutrients to escape. For this reason, peel beets after they're cooked. Watch out for beets' powerful pigments; they can stain utensils and wooden cutting boards. Microwaving retains the most nutrients. Steaming is acceptable but takes 25 to 45 minutes.

Beets have a succulent sweetness because, unlike most vegetables, they contain more sugar than starch. Beets taste great on their own, but if you'd like to enhance their delicious flavor, add a dash of salt or pepper.

BLACKBERRIES

Anyone who's experienced summer in the country knows the joys of picking berries in the hot sun. What luck that these luscious berries are good for you, too. These juicy, plump berries are low in fat and calories; in fact, a cup has approximately 70 calories. So it's easy to fill up on these flavorful berries without sabotaging your weight-loss goals.

HEALTH BENEFITS

These delightful berries are packed with pectin. By dissolving in water and forming gels that tie up blood sugar and cholesterol, pectin helps keep blood-sugar levels on an even keel.

Two thirds of blackberries' fiber is insoluble, the kind that keeps your digestive tract running smoothly. It absorbs water and swells, speeding stool and toxins through your system. Blackberries also contain a monster amount of manganese, which is important for keeping bones strong.

SELECTION AND STORAGE

Blackberries are often confused with black raspberries and related hybrids. The loganberry is a cross between a blackberry and a raspberry. The boysenberry is a cross between a blackberry, a raspberry, and a loganberry.

Indulge in blackberries in season. Though never truly economical, they are less expensive in summer. Look for berries that are glossy, plump, deep-colored, firm, and well-rounded. The darker the berries, the riper and sweeter they are. Avoid baskets of berries with juice all over the bottom—a sure sign of crushed berries. Refrigerate blackberries, but don't wash them until you're ready to eat them; otherwise they'll get moldy. Use within a day; they do not last long. For a mid-winter pick up, try freezing the berries: Arrange them in a single layer on a baking sheet, cover, and freeze. Once they are frozen, place them in an airtight container and thaw them as needed.

PREPARATION AND SERVING TIPS

Do not overhandle blackberries; their cells will break open and they will lose juice and nutrients. Wash them gently under running water, drain well, and pick through to remove stems and berries that are too soft.

Who can resist a simple bowlful of fresh berries for breakfast or a snack? You may need to sprinkle them with a little sugar if they are too tart, but go easy or you'll lose their natural low-calorie benefit. And forgo the cream—try skim milk. Served over sorbet, blackberries make a divine low-fat dessert. Don't forget the jams. Use them instead of butter or margarine on toast and muffins for the perfect fat-fighting spread.

BLACKBERRIES, FRESH
Serving Size: ¾ cup

Calories	56	Dietary Fiber	4 g
Fat	<1 g	Sodium	0 g
Saturated Fat	0 g	Vitamin C	23 mg
Cholesterol	0 mg	Manganese	1 mg
Carbohydrate	14 g	Potassium	212 mg
Protein	1 g		

Bran Cereals

You might not look forward to it, but you still pour that bowl of bran cereal every day to keep yourself regular. Little did you know your bowlful was fighting fat, too.

First, let's define what we mean by bran. Bran is simply the outer layer of any kernel of grain, where most of the fiber and nutrients reside. Here, we're just focusing on wheat bran cereals. (Oat bran is covered in the entry on oats.)

Now, back to fighting fat. Fiber, especially the insoluble kind, fills you up. It has an amazing capacity to absorb water and expand. This bulk fools your belly into thinking you've eaten a lot, so it can shut down your hunger signals.

Moreover, bran fiber requires a bit of chewing. That gives your body time to realize you're full before you shove in more. You complete the fat-fighting breakfast scene if you pour skim milk over that bowl of bran, mix in fresh fruit, and have a glass of orange juice on the side.

HEALTH BENEFITS

No other food packs such a wallop of insoluble fiber at one sitting. There's no underestimating the health boost from a daily bowl of bran cereal. Here's a chronicle.

Constipation: Eat enough insoluble fiber, such as bran, and you're practically guaranteed to avoid constipation—as long as you increase your fluid intake, too. By absorbing water, bran creates bulk, which stimulates the intestines to contract and move things along.

— Bran Cereals

Colon cancer: By increasing stool speed, bran ensures that bowel contents don't stagnate, so that means carcinogens, or cancer-causing agents, can't hang around long enough to cause trouble. And if carcinogens are present, a bulkier stool dilutes them.

Other digestive-tract conditions: A soft, swift-moving stool may prevent and ease the pain associated with many other digestive conditions, such as hemorrhoids.

All this should be enough to convince you to dig into your bowl of bran with vigor. It gets your system going in the morning while providing as much as half the suggested fiber goal of 20 to 35 grams a day (and more than half your insoluble goal of 15 to 26 grams a day).

SELECTION AND STORAGE

You don't need to swallow bran cereal as if it's medicine. Try different brands to find one you like. Bran-bud cereals provide a lot of fiber per spoonful, but flakes may be more palatable. Check labels to compare fiber and calories. Some raisin brans supply almost twice the calories. Be sure to note serving sizes; they may be very different from your usual bowlful. Compare sugar, sodium, and fat, too. But don't get paranoid about these ingredients. You're better off getting the fiber. You can make up for extra sugar, sodium, and fat at other meals.

Store opened cereals in a dry location. Once opened, they will keep for a few months before going stale. If you live in a humid environment, transfer cereals to plastic bags and refrigerate them.

FOODS THAT MAKE YOU LOSE WEIGHT

KELLOGG'S® ALL-BRAN®
Serving Size: ⅓ cup (1 oz)

Calories	70	Riboflavin	<1 mg
Fat	1 g	Niacin	5 mg
Saturated Fat	na	Vitamin B_6	<1 mg
Cholesterol	0 mg	Folic Acid	100 mcg
Carbohydrate	22 g	Copper	<1 mg
Protein	4 g	Iron	5 mg
Dietary Fiber	10 g	Magnesium	122 mg
Sodium	26 mg	Phosphorus	278 mg
Vitamin A	750 IU	Potassium	320 mg
Vitamin C	15 mg	Zinc	4 mg
Thiamin	<1 mg		

PREPARATION AND SERVING TIPS

As American breakfasts go, a bowl of bran cereal with skim milk is much, much healthier than an old-fashioned farm breakfast. While having bran for breakfast may be the best way to wake up your digestive tract, it's just as healthy as an afternoon pick-me-up or a bedtime snack. Dare to be different; top yours with nonfat yogurt instead of milk. Or sprinkle bran cereal on yogurt, salads, or cut-up fruit. Use it to coat fish or to top a tuna casserole. These are painless ways to add fat-fighting fiber to your family's menu.

BREAD, WHOLE-WHEAT

You probably know whole wheat is the best type of wheat, but just because your bread is brown doesn't mean it's whole wheat. Even if the label proudly boasts "wheat" bread and lists "wheat flour" as the first ingredient, your bread may still not be whole wheat. Confused?

"Wheat" simply refers to the grain the flour comes from. Anything made with the flour from wheat—even refined white bread—can be called "wheat" and can list "wheat flour" as an ingredient. (The brown color often comes from caramel coloring.) Are manufacturers lying to consumers? No. But are their labeling practices misleading? We think so. Being informed will guard you from being misled. Learning the facts will help you choose the right bread.

Mistakenly, many people still think bread is fattening. On the contrary, bread can be the best fat-fighting friend in your diet. Bread is naturally low in fat and can be high in fiber. Because it is so versatile, you can easily eat many servings a day in place of other more fattening foods. As long as you don't pile on fatty spreads or fillings, bread can help you lose weight. In fact, studies have proved that people who eat 8 to 12 slices of bread a day still lose weight as long as their total diet is low in fat and calories. The trick is keeping yourself from slathering that hearty bread with butter or margarine.

HEALTH BENEFITS

Whole-wheat bread, in particular, is good for you for a number of reasons. It's high in complex carbohydrates, low in fat, a source of protein, and a storehouse of nutrients and fiber—a microcosm of what your diet should be.

To understand what's so special about whole wheat in particular, you need to understand the structure of wheat grain. There are three basic layers to the grain—endosperm, germ, and bran. When whole-wheat flour is milled (refined) to make white bread, the germ and outer bran layer are removed, leaving only the inner endosperm. Unfortunately, more than half the fiber of wheat is in that bran and germ, along with almost three quarters of the vitamins and minerals. Besides nutrients, the milling process also removes nonnutrient components—phytoestrogens, phenolic acids, oryzanol, and tannins—that may have health benefits, like reducing your risk of cancer.

What milling removes, manufacturers try to put back in. Lost B vitamins—thiamin, riboflavin, niacin—and iron are added back to form enriched bread products. Many other nutrients, especially minerals and fiber, don't get added back. So if you eat white bread, you're definitely missing a fiber opportunity.

SELECTION AND STORAGE

The key to buying whole-wheat bread is to be sure it says "100% whole wheat." Unless you read the word "whole," you're not getting all the goodness of the bran and germ of the wheat berry.

What about whole-grain or multigrain breads? They sound and look healthy, but refined wheat flour still may be the primary ingredient. Your only defense against being fooled is to read labels carefully. If you want 100 percent whole wheat, whole wheat should be the only grain listed. If you like the taste of multigrain breads, pick one that lists whole wheat first in the list of ingredients. Then you know it's the predominant grain.

Cracked-wheat breads are not always 100 percent whole cracked wheat. Again, check the label. Pumpernickel bread looks hearty but is really just a form of rye bread with caramel or molasses added. Both rye and pumpernickel breads are usually made from refined rye flour with the bran and germ removed, because breads made with 100 percent rye grain are too dense. If you can find it, look for rye bread made from "unbolted" rye and whole wheat.

Check the expiration date of the bread you buy. Many whole-wheat breads lack preservatives that prolong freshness. To prevent bread from going stale, only leave out at room temperature as much as you'll eat in a day or two, keeping it tightly closed in a plastic bag. Freeze the rest. Take out slices as you need them; they'll defrost quickly at room temperature. Don't refrigerate your bread—it only goes stale faster.

If you see mold on bread, throw out the entire loaf, as well as the bag itself. Mold usually starts as a whitish bloom. You can't salvage bread that's moldy, because mold spores spread quickly throughout soft foods. Do not even smell the inside of the bag; you may inhale mold spores.

PREPARATION AND SERVING TIPS

You don't have to resort to stalking the aisles and investigating ingredient labels for the perfect loaf of bread. You can make it yourself. Nothing could be fresher or taste better. Not knowing how to bake bread or not having the time are no longer excuses if you have a bread-making machine. For per-

WHOLE-WHEAT BREAD
Serving Size: 1 slice

Calories	61	Thiamin	<1 mg
Fat	1 g	Niacin	1 mg
Saturated Fat	na	Chromium	14 mcg
Cholesterol	0 mg	Copper	<1 mg
Carbohydrate	11 g	Iron	1 mg
Protein	2 g	Magnesium	23 mg
Dietary Fiber	2 g	Manganese	<1 mg
Sodium	159 mg		

fect rising, look for whole-wheat bread flour, which contains more gluten. Add nonfat dry milk powder for extra protein and calcium. Add wheat germ for extra fiber and a hefty dose of nutrients.

BROCCOLI

Best nutritious vegetable? Broccoli wins hands down. Eat it raw or cooked—as long as you don't cover it with cheese sauce, it can be part of your fat-fighting repertoire. You simply can't get a bigger dose of more nutrients from any other vegetable, especially for so few calories. That's key for those who are trying to lose weight; it's hard to meet nutrient needs when you're eating very-low-calorie foods.

HEALTH BENEFITS

Broccoli's noteworthy nutrients include vitamin C, vitamin A (mostly as beta-carotene), folic acid, calcium, and fiber. While the calcium content of one serving doesn't equal that of a glass of milk, broccoli is an important calcium source for those who don't consume dairy products. Calcium does more than build strong bones. Research shows that this mineral may play a role in the control of high blood pressure, and it may work to prevent colon cancer.

Beta-carotene and vitamin C are important antioxidants that have been linked to a reduced risk of numerous conditions, including cataracts, heart disease, and several cancers.

Broccoli is a fiber find. Not only is it a rich source, but half of its fiber is insoluble and half is soluble, helping to meet your needs for both types of fiber.

But the story doesn't end with broccoli's rich array of nutrients. Broccoli provides a health bonus in the form of protective substances that may shield you from disease. Botanically, broccoli belongs to the cabbage family, collectively known as cruciferous vegetables. Health organizations have singled out cruciferous vegetables as must-have foods, recommending we eat them several times a week. Why? They are linked to lower rates of cancer. Like all cruciferous vegetables, broccoli naturally contains two important phytochemicals—indoles and isothiocyanates. Not long ago, researchers at Johns Hopkins University School of Medicine in Baltimore isolated from broccoli an isothiocyanate, called sulforaphane, that increases the activity of a group of enzymes in our bodies that squelch cancer-causing agents.

SELECTION AND STORAGE

Look for broccoli that's dark green or even purplish-green, but not yellow. Florets should be compact and of even color; leaves should not be wilted; and stalks should not be fat and woody. The greener it is, the more beta-carotene it has.

Keep broccoli cold. At room temperature, the sugar in broccoli is converted into a fiber called lignin, which is woody and fibrous. Store unwashed broccoli in your refrigerator's crisper drawer, in a plastic bag. Don't completely seal the bag, but make sure it is tight. Use within a few days.

PREPARATION AND SERVING TIPS

Wash broccoli just before using. Cut off as much of the stems as you like; they contain fewer nutrients than the florets anyway. Steaming is the best way to cook broccoli because many nutrients are lost when it's boiled. Preventing broccoli's unpleasant odor is easy—don't use an aluminum pan and don't overcook it. Steam only until crisp-tender, while stalks are still bright green; five minutes is plenty. Try this trick:

Broccoli, Fresh, Cooked
Serving Size: ½ cup chopped

Calories	23	Vitamin C	49 mg
Fat	<1 g	Riboflavin	1 mg
Saturated Fat	0 g	Vitamin B6	1 mg
Cholesterol	0 mg	Folic Acid	53 mcg
Carbohydrate	4 g	Calcium	89 mg
Protein	2 g	Iron	1 mg
Dietary Fiber	2 g	Magnesium	47 mg
Sodium	8 mg	Manganese	1 mg
Vitamin A	1,099 IU		

Make one or two cuts through the stems before cooking. This helps the stems cook as fast as the tops.

When serving broccoli, skip the cheese sauce. Keep it simple; add a squeeze of lemon and a dusting of cracked pepper.

Broccoli florets can boost the nutrition, flavor, and color of any stir-fry dish. Raw broccoli tossed into salads boosts the nutrition of a midday meal.

Served raw, broccoli is a great finger food. Children love it this way, perhaps because the flavor isn't as strong, or maybe just because it's fun. Double the fun by giving them a dipping sauce to dunk it in, like fat-free ranch dressing.

BRUSSELS SPROUTS

No one knows the origin of brussels sprouts, though it's logical to assume they originated in Belgium. Like all vegetables, brussels sprouts are naturally low in fat. But unlike most vegetables, brussels sprouts are rather high in protein, accounting for more than a quarter of their calories. Although the protein is incomplete—it doesn't provide the full spectrum of essential amino acids—it can be made complete with whole grains. This means you can skip a fattier source of protein, like meat, and rely on a meal of brussels sprouts and grains now and again—truly a fat fighter.

HEALTH BENEFITS

Brussels sprouts are also very high in fiber, and they belong to the disease-fighting cabbage family. Indeed, they look like miniature cabbages. Like broccoli and cabbage—fellow cruciferous vegetables—brussels sprouts may protect against cancer with their indole, a phytochemical. They are also particularly rich in vitamin C, another anti-cancer agent.

SELECTION AND STORAGE

Fresh brussels sprouts shine in fall and winter. Look for a pronounced green color and tight, compact, firm heads. The fewer the yellowed, wilted, or loose leaves the better.

You're better off choosing smaller heads; they're more tender and flavorful. Pick ones of similar size so they cook evenly. Stored in the refrigerator in the cardboard container they came in or kept in a plastic bag, loosely closed, they'll last a week or two.

BRUSSELS SPROUTS, FRESH, COOKED
Serving Size: ½ cup

Calories	30	Sodium	17 mg
Fat	<1 g	Vitamin A	561 IU
Saturated Fat	0 g	Vitamin C	48 mg
Cholesterol	0 mg	Folic Acid	47 mcg
Carbohydrate	7 g	Iron	1 mg
Protein	2 g	Manganese	<1 mg
Dietary Fiber	4 g	Potassium	257 mg

PREPARATION AND SERVING TIPS

Dunk sprouts in ice water to debug them. Then rinse them under running water. Pull off loose or wilted leaves; trim the stem ends a little. Cut an "X" in the bottoms, so the insides cook at the same rate as the leaves. Steaming is your best bet. The sprouts will stay intact, odor will be minimized, and you'll preserve more nutrients than you would if you boiled them.

As with broccoli and cabbage, the odor becomes most pronounced when overcooked. Brussels sprouts also lose valuable vitamin C when overcooked. So don't be afraid to leave your sprouts a bit on the crisp side. As soon as you can barely prick them with a fork they're done—about 7 to 14 minutes, depending on size.

Brussels sprouts are delicious served with just a squeeze of lemon. For more flavor, try a mustard sauce.

BUCKWHEAT

There's more to buckwheat than flapjacks. Eastern Europeans know roasted buckwheat groats as kasha and eat it like porridge. Despite its name, buckwheat is not a type of wheat—nor is it related to wheat. Buckwheat isn't even a grain; it's the fruit of a plant that's related to rhubarb.

HEALTH BENEFITS

Buckwheat contains more protein than true grains and is not deficient in the amino acid lysine as most grains are, so the protein is more nutritionally complete. That makes it a particularly good choice for vegetarians. It's an excellent source of magnesium, a boon to your blood pressure. Presumably, it's relatively rich in fiber, but exact values aren't available.

SELECTION AND STORAGE

Most of our buckwheat comes from New York and carries a premium price, because so few farmers grow it. Look for it in health-food stores or mail-order catalogs. In larger cities, check stores in Russian or Slavic neighborhoods.

Buckwheat is sold as groats, grits, or flour. Groats are pale kernels without the hard, inedible outer shell. You can buy them whole or cracked into coarse, medium, or fine grinds. Roasted groats—kasha—are dark kernels. Very finely cracked unroasted groats are buckwheat grits. They can be found as a hot cereal—sometimes labeled "cream of buckwheat." Buckwheat flour is also available, in light and dark versions. The darker type contains more of the hull, therefore more fiber and nutrients, and imparts a stronger flavor.

— BUCKWHEAT

Keep buckwheat in a well-sealed container in a cool, dark location. At room temperature, it is more susceptible to turning rancid than are true grains, especially in warm climates. Keep it in the refrigerator or freezer.

PREPARATION AND SERVING TIPS

Take advantage of buckwheat's intense, nutty flavor. If you don't care for kasha plain, mix it in with pasta, grains, potatoes, or vegetables—especially winter vegetables. It makes a hearty, flavorful meal. For pilafs, stuffing, and soups, use whole kasha. Save the medium and fine grinds for cereals.

To cook: Combine ½ cup whole groats with a cup of water and simmer for 15 minutes. It will triple in volume. Or combine ½ cup of cracked kasha with 2½ cups of liquid and cook for 12 minutes, to yield 2 cups.

Buckwheat flour is superb for pancakes, but don't try making bread with it; it doesn't work because it contains no gluten. But you can add ¼ to ½ cup of buckwheat flour into a recipe for bread, as long as the primary grain is wheat or another high-gluten grain.

BUCKWHEAT GROATS, ROASTED, COOKED (KASHA)
Serving Size: ½ cup

Calories................91	Cholesterol................0
Protein ....3.4 g	Dietary Fiber ....na
Carbohydrate .....19.7 g	Sodium................4 mg
Fat........................0.6 g	Iron....................0.8 mg
Saturated..........0.1 g	Magnesium ....51 mg

FOODS THAT MAKE YOU LOSE WEIGHT

BULGUR

This Middle Eastern staple sounds more exotic than it is; bulgur is what's left after wheat kernels have been steamed, dried, and crushed. This cereal grain has been a food staple for years because it offers an inexpensive source of low-fat protein, making it a wonderfully nutritious addition to your low-fat meal plan.

HEALTH BENEFITS

Bulgur doesn't lose much from its minimal processing; it remains high in protein and minerals. That means it's an ideal foundation for meals, allowing you to skip higher-fat protein sources, like meat.

Bulgur is also a standout in terms of its fiber content, just like whole wheat, and can help keep your digestive tract healthy as a result. The insoluble fiber it contains absorbs water, promoting faster elimination of waste, which prevents the formation of an environment that promotes the development of carcinogens.

SELECTION AND STORAGE

You may need to visit a health-food store to find bulgur. It's available in three grinds—coarse, medium, and fine. Coarse bulgur is used to make pilaf or stuffing. Medium-grind bulgur is used in cereals. The finest grind of bulgur is suited to the popular cold Middle Eastern salad called tabbouleh. Store bulgur in a screw-top glass jar in the refrigerator; it will keep for months.

— BULGUR

PREPARATION AND SERVING TIPS

Because bulgur is already partially cooked, little time is needed for preparation: Combine a half cup of bulgur with one cup of liquid and simmer for 15 minutes. Let stand for another ten minutes. Fluff with a fork. It triples in volume.

For cold salads, soak bulgur before using: Pour boiling water over bulgur, in a three-to-one ratio. Soak for 30 to 40 minutes. Drain away excess water. If you like your bulgur chewier, let it sit longer to absorb more water.

Bulgur is used like rice in Mediterranean countries. In fact, you can use bulgur in place of rice in most recipes. Bulgur lends its nutty flavor to whatever it is combined with, allowing you to use it as a main ingredient, thus cutting back on fattier foods.

BULGUR, COOKED
Serving Size: ½ cup

Calories....................76	Dietary Fiber..............4 g
Fat............................<1 g	Sodium.......................5 mg
Saturated Fat.........0 g	Iron.............................1 mg
Cholesterol.................0 mg	Magnesium..............29 mg
Carbohydrate...........17 g	Manganese................1 mg
Protein........................3 g	

CABBAGE

Cabbage is at the head of the cruciferous vegetable family. But it's a vegetable that few people appreciate. Though strong-flavored, it's this feature that makes you less likely to miss the flavor of fat in your diet. In fact, cabbage is a dieter's friend, with among the fewest calories and least fat of any vegetable.

HEALTH BENEFITS

From green cabbage you'll enjoy a fiber boost and a respectable amount of vitamin C. Two types of cabbage, savoy and bok choy, provide beta-carotene—an antioxidant that battles cancer and heart disease. For vegetarians, bok choy is an important source of calcium, which may help prevent osteoporosis and aid in controlling blood pressure.

The phytochemicals in cabbage, called indoles, are also being studied for their ability to convert estradiol, an estrogenlike hormone that may play a role in the development of breast cancer, into a safer form of estrogen—powerful incentives to add cabbage to your diet.

SELECTION AND STORAGE

There are literally hundreds of varieties of cabbage. Green cabbage is the most familiar kind, with Danish, domestic, and pointed being the top three picks of the cabbage family. All sport the familiar pale green, compact head; are similar nutritionally; and shine in fiber. Red cabbage, a cousin of the green, has a bit more vitamin C, but the most nutritious is savoy cabbage, which has a pretty, dark-green, round head that's loose, ruffly, and prominently "veined." It is much higher in beta-carotene—about ten times more—than green or red cabbage. Napa cabbage, also known as celery cabbage or pe-tsai, is often incorrectly called Chinese cabbage. Nutritionally, it's equivalent to green cabbage.

Bok choy, or pak-choi, is true Chinese cabbage. As its dark green color suggests, it's rich in beta-carotene. It's also a good source of potassium and a particularly well-absorbed nondairy source of calcium, providing about ten percent of a day's requirement. It only falls short in the fiber category.

When choosing green and red cabbage, pick a tight, compact head that feels heavy for its size. It should look crisp and fresh, with few loose leaves. Leafy varieties should be green, with stems that are firm, not limp.

Store whole heads of cabbage in the crisper drawer of your refrigerator. If uncut, compact heads keep for a couple of weeks. Leafy varieties should be used within a few days.

Preparation and Serving Tips

Discard outer leaves if loose or limp, cut into quarters, then wash. When cooking quarters, leave the core in as this prevents the leaves from tearing apart. If shredding cabbage for coleslaw, core the cabbage first. But don't shred ahead of time; once you do, enzymes begin destroying vitamin C.

Forget old-fashioned corned beef and cabbage recipes. More nutrients will be preserved and the cabbage will taste better if it is cooked only until slightly tender, but still crisp—about 10 to 12 minutes for wedges, five minutes if shredded. Red cabbage takes a few minutes more; leafy varieties cook faster.

GREEN CABBAGE, FRESH, COOKED
Serving Size: ½ cup chopped

Calories	16	Protein	1 g
Fat	<1 g	Dietary Fiber	3 g
Saturated Fat	0 g	Sodium	5 mg
Cholesterol	0 mg	Vitamin C	18 mg
Carbohydrate	4 g		

BOK CHOY, FRESH, COOKED
Serving Size: ½ cup chopped

Calories	10	Sodium	29 mg
Fat	<1 g	Vitamin A	2,183 IU
Saturated Fat	0 g	Vitamin C	22 mg
Cholesterol	0 mg	Calcium	79 mg
Carbohydrate	2 g	Iron	1 mg
Protein	1 g	Potassium	315 mg
Dietary Fiber	1 g		

To solve cabbage's notorious stink problem, steam it in a small amount of water for a short time and do not cook it in an aluminum pan. Uncover briefly, shortly after cooking begins, to release the sulfur smell.

Combine red and green cabbage for a more interesting cole slaw. Keep the fat down with a dressing of nonfat yogurt laced with poppy seeds. Bok choy and napa cabbage work well in stir-fry dishes. Savoy is perfect for stuffing. In place of the meat in traditional stuffed-cabbage recipes, use a grain like bulgur, quinoa, or buckwheat.

CARROTS

If you don't have a bag of carrots sitting in your refrigerator, you should—they're anything but ordinary when it comes to nutrition. Carrots contain an uncommon amount of beta-carotene. And they can masquerade as a fat substitute by serving as a thickener in soups, sauces, casseroles, and quick breads. Because of its terrific replacement qualities, you don't have to add any cream, or fat for that matter, to cream of carrot soup. In fact, their numerous health benefits call for amending that well-known saying to: A carrot a day keeps the doctor away.

HEALTH BENEFITS

One of carrots' fat-fighting features is their respectable fiber content, half of which is the soluble fiber calcium pectate. Soluble fiber may help lower blood-cholesterol levels by binding with and eliminating bile acids, triggering cholesterol to be drawn out of the bloodstream to make more bile acids.

Carrots have few rivals when it comes to beta-carotene. A mere half-cup serving of cooked carrots packs a walloping four times the RDA of vitamin A in the form of protective beta-carotene. One raw carrot supposedly contains as much, though it's not clear if all of it's usable by your body. The strongest evidence for beta-carotene's protective antioxidant effect is against lung tumors (though avoiding tobacco is still your best defense), but beta-carotene may also ward off cancers of the stomach, cervix, uterus, and oral cavity.

The National Cancer Institute is studying the whole family of umbelliferous foods, of which carrots are a member, for protective effects. Recent research results from Harvard University suggest that people who eat more than five carrots a week are much less likely to suffer a stroke than those who eat only one carrot a month.

Finally, like Mom said, carrots do help your eyes. The retina of the eye needs vitamin A to function; a deficiency of vitamin A causes night blindness. Though extra vitamin A won't help you see better, its antioxidant properties may help prevent cataracts.

SELECTION AND STORAGE

Look for firm carrots with bright orange color and smooth skin. Avoid carrots if they are limp or black near the tops; they're not fresh. Choose medium-sized ones that taper at the ends. Thicker ones taste tough. In general, early carrots are more tender but less sweet than larger, mature carrots.

Clip greens as soon as you are home to avoid moisture loss. Store greens and carrots separately in perforated plastic bags in your refrigerator's crisper drawer. Carrots keep for a few weeks; greens last only a few days.

PREPARATION AND SERVING TIPS

Thoroughly wash and scrub carrots to remove soil contaminants. Being root vegetables, carrots tend to end up with more pesticide residues than nonroot vegetables. You can get rid of much of it by peeling the outer layer and by cutting off and discarding one-quarter inch off the fat end.

CARROTS, FRESH, COOKED
Serving Size: ½ cup chopped

Calories	35	Dietary Fiber	2 g
Fat	<1 g	Sodium	52 mg
Saturated Fat	0 g	Vitamin A	19,152 IU
Cholesterol	0 mg	Vitamin B6	<1 mg
Carbohydrate	8 g	Manganese	<1 mg
Protein	1 g	Potassium	177 mg

Carrots are a great raw snack, of course. But their true sweet flavor shines through when cooked. Very little nutritional value is lost in cooking, unless you overcook them until mushy. In fact, the nutrients in lightly cooked carrots are more usable by your body than those in raw carrots, because cooking breaks down their tough cell walls, which releases beta-carotene.

Steaming is your best bet for cooking carrots. Take advantage of the fact that most children love carrots, raw or cooked. But avoid serving coin-shaped slices to young children; they can choke on them. Cut them into quarters or julienne strips.

For that fat-free carrot soup mentioned above, use carrots and leeks for thickening. Add onions, chicken stock, white pepper, and you're in business. In fact, the soluble fiber in carrots can add thickness to lots of foods, taking the place of fattening butter and cream. The stronger the flavor of the soup or sauce, the more it will hide the carrot flavor. You can even use carrots when baking, as long as you puree them.

CAULIFLOWER

Cauliflower, one of several cruciferous vegetables, is an ideal fat-fighting companion for meatless meals. Its strong flavor allows it to stand alone without meat or other fatty foods. And if you're really hungry, raw cauliflower makes a wonderful snack. Because it's extra crunchy, cauliflower takes longer to chew, giving your body time to realize you're full before you eat yourself out of house and home.

HEALTH BENEFITS

After citrus fruits, cauliflower is your next best natural source of vitamin C, an antioxidant that appears to help combat cancer. It's also an important warrior in the continuous battle our bodies wage against infection. Cauliflower is also notable for its fiber, folic acid, and potassium contents, proving it's more nutritious than its white appearance would have you believe. Cauliflower may also be a natural cancer fighter. It contains phytochemicals, called indoles, that may stimulate enzymes that block cancer growth.

SELECTION AND STORAGE

Though cauliflower is available year-round, it's more reasonably priced in season—fall and winter. Look for creamy white heads with compact florets. Brown patches and opened florets are signs of aging.

Store unwashed, uncut cauliflower loosely wrapped in a plastic bag in your refrigerator's crisper drawer. Keep upright to prevent moisture from collecting on the surface. It will keep two to five days.

Cauliflower, Fresh, Cooked
Serving Size: ½ cup

Calories....................15	Dietary Fiber ....1 g
Fat..........................<1 g	Sodium.......................4 mg
Saturated Fat.........0 g	Vitamin C ....34 mg
Cholesterol................0 mg	Folic Acid ....32 mcg
Carbohydrate ....3 g	Potassium ....200 mg
Protein........................1 g	

PREPARATION AND SERVING TIPS

Remove outer leaves, break off florets, trim brown spots, and wash them under running water. Cauliflower serves up well both raw and cooked. Raw, its flavor is less intense and more acceptable to children. Let them dip it into fat-free dressing.

Steam cauliflower, but don't overcook it. Overcooking destroys its vitamin C and folic acid. Moreover, overcooking gives cauliflower a bitter, pungent flavor. To prevent this, steam it in a nonaluminum pan over a small amount of water, until a fork barely pierces a floret—about five minutes. Remove the cover soon after cooking begins to release odoriferous sulfur compounds.

Although cheese sauces are popular over cauliflower, they add a hefty dose of fat and calories. Why ruin a good thing? Better to serve cauliflower plain or with a little dill weed. For a low-fat, meatless meal, add cauliflower, broccoli, and carrots to homemade tomato sauce; simmer for 15 minutes, then enjoy over hot pasta.

CORN

Corn is a low-fat complex carbohydrate that deserves a regular place on any healthy table. Unfortunately, as with many other naturally low-fat foods, the American tendency is to smother corn-on-the-cob with butter. But these high-fiber, fat-fighting kernels of goodness are better left alone. Because corn is hearty and satisfying, it can curb your appetite for high-fat foods.

HEALTH BENEFITS

This popular food is high in fiber. In fact, it's notoriously hard to digest. But its insoluble fiber is tops at tackling common digestive ailments (like constipation and hemorrhoids) by absorbing water, which swells the stool and speeds its movement.

Corn is a surprising source of several vitamins, including folic acid, niacin, and vitamin C. The folic acid in corn is now known to be an important factor in preventing neural-tube birth defects. It's just as important in preventing heart disease, according to new studies that show folic acid can prevent a buildup of homocysteine, an amino acid, in the body. Long-term elevation of homocysteine has been linked to higher rates of heart disease; folic acid helps break it down.

SELECTION AND STORAGE

End-of-summer corn is by far the best ear in town. Although you can find good-tasting corn year-round, many out-of-season ears aren't worth eating. When buying fresh corn, be sure

CORN, YELLOW OR WHITE
Serving Size: 1 ear

Calories	83	Dietary Fiber	3 g
Fat	1 g	Sodium	13 mg
Saturated Fat	<1 g	Vitamin C	5 mg
Cholesterol	0 mg	Folic Acid	36 mcg
Carbohydrate	19 g	Niacin	1 mg
Protein	3 g	Potassium	192 mg

it was delivered in cold storage—as temperatures rise, the natural sugar in corn turns to starch, and the corn loses some sweetness. Corn is best eaten within a day or two of picking.

Corn husks should be green and have visible kernels that are plump and tightly packed on the cob. To test freshness, pop a kernel with your fingernail. The liquid that spurts out should be milky colored. If not, the corn is either immature or overripe. Once home, refrigerate corn immediately.

PREPARATION AND SERVING TIPS

Boiling is the traditional method for preparing corn-on-the-cob, though grilling, steaming, and even microwaving will get the job done. A couple of notes about boiling: Adding salt to the water toughens corn; adding sugar isn't necessary; overcooking toughens kernels. Cook for the shortest amount of time possible—about five minutes.

Though you may be tempted to slather on butter or margarine, keep in mind that each pat you add contributes about five unnecessary grams of fat to your diet. Instead, sprinkle with a favorite herb or fresh-squeezed lemon juice.

DATES

Dates are among the most ancient of fruits, growing along the Nile as early as the fifth century B.C. Perhaps the Egyptians knew dates' sweetness hid a bounty of nutrients. Dates are nuggets of nutrition that satisfy a sweet tooth, making them ideal snacks to stave off hunger. True, dates provide more calories than most fruits, but they are practically fat-free.

HEALTH BENEFITS

Loaded with fiber—both soluble and insoluble—dates are able to fill you up and keep your bowel habits regular. They are an excellent source of potassium and provide numerous other important vitamins and minerals—quite a powerhouse packed in a tiny, portable package.

SELECTION AND STORAGE

Most supermarkets stock fresh dates; you may have to visit a health-food store to find dried dates. For both types look for plump fruit with unbroken, smoothly wrinkled skins. Avoid dates that smell bad or have hardened sugar crystals on their skins.

Packaged dates are available pitted, unpitted, or chopped. Dried dates keep for up to a year in the refrigerator. Fresh dates should be refrigerated in tightly sealed containers; they'll keep up to eight months. If stored in the kitchen cabinet, they'll stay fresh for about a month.

If dates dry out, they can be "plumped" with a little warm water, fruit juice, or for fancier dishes, your favorite liqueur.

— DATES

Don't store dates near strongly flavored items such as garlic; they tend to absorb outside odors.

PREPARATION AND SERVING TIPS

Dates are great on their own, but for an extra-special treat, try stuffing them with whole almonds or chopped pieces of walnuts or pecans. For a spicy twist, tuck in a piece of crystallized gingerroot.

Adding dates to home-baked breads, cakes, muffins, and cookies adds richness and nutrition to otherwise ordinary recipes. And the natural moisture of dates adds to the quality of the final product. Dates work well in fruit compotes, salads, and desserts. Chopped or slivered, dates can even be sprinkled on side dishes like rice, couscous, or vegetables.

To slice or chop dates, chill them first; the colder they are, the easier they are to slice.

DATES, DRIED
Serving Size: 10 dates

Calories	228	Pantothenic Acid	1 mg
Fat	<1 g	Vitamin B_6	<1 mg
Saturated Fat	na	Calcium	27 mg
Cholesterol	0 mg	Copper	<1 mg
Carbohydrate	61 g	Iron	1 mg
Protein	2 g	Magnesium	29 mg
Dietary Fiber	6 g	Manganese	<1 mg
Sodium	2 mg	Potassium	541 mg
Niacin	2 mg		

FISH

Fish is a delicacy not to be missed. It's a fabulous addition to any healthful diet because its low fat content (generally 20 percent or less of total calories) makes it the perfect protein substitute for fatty cuts of beef and pork. Even shellfish is low in fat and isn't as high in cholesterol as many believe.

HEALTH BENEFITS

Although fish is lean, it does contain some oil. Known as omega-3 fatty acids, these fish oils are thought to offer some amazing health benefits, such as helping to prevent heart disease and cancer, treating psoriasis and arthritis, and relieving the agony of migraine headaches. Fatty fish tend to have more omega-3s than leaner fish, but even "fatty" fish contain less fat than lean beef or chicken.

Even canned fish like tuna, sardines, and salmon have omega-3s, and sardines and salmon, when eaten bones and all, pack your meal with an ample amount of good-for-your-bones calcium, too.

SELECTION AND STORAGE

When buying fresh fish, always smell it. If you detect a "fishy" odor, don't buy it. Whether you buy whole fish, fish fillets, or steaks, the fish should be firm to the touch. The scales should be shiny and clean, not slimy. Check the eyes; they should be clear, not cloudy and bulging, not sunken. Fish fillets and steaks should be moist. If they look dried or curled around the edges they probably aren't fresh.

It's best to cook fresh fish the same day you buy it. (Fish generally spoils faster than beef or chicken, and whole fish generally keeps better than steaks or fillets.) But it will keep in the refrigerator overnight if you store it in an airtight container over a bowl of ice.

If you need to keep it longer than a day, freeze it. The quality of thawed, frozen fish is better when it freezes quickly, so freeze whole fish only if it weighs two pounds or less; larger fish should be cut into pieces, steaks, or fillets to ensure a quick freeze. Lean fish will keep in the freezer for up to six months—three months for fatty fish.

When buying most shellfish—clams, oysters, lobsters, crabs and crayfish—it's imperative they still be alive. Live lobsters and crabs are easy to spot. Clams and oysters are trickier though; you must be sure the shell is closed tightly or closes when you tap the shell.

Fish and shellfish have been dogged by safety questions, including those arising from man-made contaminants. Oysters and clams carry a particular risk of passing on diseases such as hepatitis or Norwalk-like viruses if eaten raw. New

COHO SALMON
Serving Size: 3 oz, cooked

Calories 157	Protein......................23 g
Fat.............................6 g	Dietary Fiber ....0 g
Saturated Fat.........1 g	Sodium......................50 mg
Cholesterol...............42 mg	Potassium ....454 mg
Carbohydrate ....0 g	

Snapper

Serving Size: 3 oz, cooked

Calories	109	Protein	22 g
Fat	2 g	Dietary Fiber	0 g
Saturated Fat	<1 g	Sodium	48 mg
Cholesterol	40 mg	Magnesium	31 mg
Carbohydrate	0 g	Potassium	444 mg

research suggests even typical cooking may not be enough to kill all bacterial threats. Pesticides, mercury, and chemicals like PCB sometimes find their way into fish. Though fatty fish is richer in omega-3s, they're also more likely to harbor environmental contaminants.

Here are precautions you can take to reduce the odds of eating contaminated fish:

• Eat fish from a variety of sources.

• Opt for open ocean fish and farmed fish over freshwater fish; they are less likely to harbor toxins.

• Eat smaller, young fish. Older fish are more likely to have accumulated chemicals in their fatty tissues.

• Before you fish, check your own state's advisories about which waters are unsafe for fishing. Try the Department of Public Health or the Department of Environmental Conservation.

• Don't make a habit of eating the fish you catch for sport if you fish in the same area over and over again.

• Avoid swordfish; it may be contaminated with mercury.

Preparation and Serving Tips

For the uninitiated, fish is most perplexing to prepare. But the number one rule is: Preserve moistness. That means avoiding direct heat, especially when preparing low-fat varieties of fish; you'll get the best results if you use moist-heat methods such as poaching, steaming, or baking with vegetables or in a sauce. Dry-heat methods such as baking, broiling, and grilling work well for fattier fish.

Fish cooks fast, so it's easy to overcook it. You can tell fish is done when it looks opaque and the flesh just begins to flake with the touch of a fork. If it falls apart when you touch it, it's too late; the fish is overdone. The general rule of thumb for cooking fish is to cook eight to ten minutes per inch of thickness, measured at the fish's thickest point.

For fish soups, stews, and chowders, use lean fish. An oily fish will overpower the flavor of the broth. Citrus juices enhance the natural flavor of fish. Lemon, lime, or orange juice complements almost any kind of fish. Some favorite fish seasonings are dill, tarragon, basil, paprika, parsley, and thyme.

GARLIC

Through the centuries, garlic has been both reviled and revered for its qualities. Today, the gossip about garlic and its apparent disease-preventing potential has reached a fevered pitch. For garlic lovers, that's good news; adding garlic to dishes can make up for bland low-fat preparations. Once you learn to appreciate its pungency, most anything tastes better with garlic. And once you learn its possible health benefits, you may learn to love it.

HEALTH BENEFITS

The list of health benefits just seems to grow and grow. From preventing heart disease and cancer to fighting off infections, researchers are finding encouraging results with garlic. Behind all the grandiose claims are the compounds that give garlic its biting flavor. The chief health-promoting "ingredients" are allicin and diallyl sulfide, sulfur-containing compounds. The biggest question surrounding them is whether their disease-preventing abilities remain intact once cooked. No one really knows for sure. But it's believed that at least some health benefits survive cooking.

Garlic has been found to lower levels of LDL cholesterol, the "bad" cholesterol, and raise HDL cholesterol, the "good" cholesterol. It may also help to dissolve clots that can lead to heart attacks and strokes.

Garlic has also been found to inhibit the growth of, or even kill, several kinds of bacteria, including *Staphylococcus* and *Salmonella*, as well as many fungi and yeast.

— Garlic

Animal studies have found that garlic helps prevent colon, lung, and esophageal cancers. How much is enough? No one knows. In many studies, garlic extracts were used, making it impossible to translate into a practical prescription for better health.

SELECTION AND STORAGE

Most varieties of garlic have the same characteristic pungent odor and bite. Pink-skinned garlic tastes a little sweeter and keeps longer than white garlic. Elephant garlic, a large-clove variety, is milder in flavor than regular garlic. But most varieties can be used interchangeably in recipes.

Opt for loose garlic if you can find it. It's easier to check the quality of what you're getting than with those hiding behind cellophane. Its appearance can clue you in to its freshness; paper-white skins are your best bet. Then pick up the garlic; choose a head that is firm to the touch with no visible damp or brown spots.

Don't expect the flavor of garlic powder to mimic fresh garlic. Much of the flavor is processed out. Garlic powder, however, does retain large amounts of active components. Garlic salt, of course, contains large amounts of sodium—as much as 900 milligrams per teaspoon.

Store garlic in a cool, dark, dry spot. If you don't use it regularly, check it occasionally to be sure it's usable. Garlic may last only a few weeks or a few months. If one or two cloves have gone bad, remove them, but don't nick remaining cloves; any skin punctures will hasten the demise of what's left. If garlic begins to sprout, it's still okay to use, but it may have a milder flavor.

Garlic

Serving Size: 3 cloves

Calories	13	Carbohydrate	3 g
Fat	1 g	Protein	1 g
Saturated Fat	0 g	Dietary Fiber	<1 g
Cholesterol	0 mg	Sodium	2 mg

PREPARATION AND SERVING TIPS

Garlic squeezed through a garlic press is ten times stronger in flavor than garlic minced with a knife, so use pressed garlic when you want full-force flavor to come through; use minced when you want to curtail it; and for a buttery flavor, bake whole cloves until tender. The longer the garlic is cooked, the more mild the flavor.

For just a delicate touch of garlic in salads, rub the bottom of the salad bowl with a cut clove before adding the salad greens. For more flavor, add freshly crushed garlic to the salad.

You can make your own version of fat-free garlic bread by warming a loaf of bread, spreading the inside with a fresh cut clove of garlic, then toasting the loaf under the broiler. You'll get a teaser of garlic without all the fat.

Chew on fresh parsley, fresh mint, or citrus peel to neutralize the pungent aroma garlic leaves on your breath—a common complaint among garlic lovers. This doesn't work for everyone, but it just might help you.

GRAPEFRUIT

No, grapefruit is not a calorie-free fruit, as some diets would have you believe. Despite its reputation as a "fat-burner," grapefruit has no special ability to burn away excess fat. But it is low in calories with essentially no fat, and its soluble fiber content is decent enough to fill you up, discouraging you from overeating. So yes, grapefruit can help you lose weight, just not as easily as some would say. And it's nutritious, to boot. Grapefruit is a tart-tasting fruit not everyone enjoys. But for those who do, grapefruit offers a lot of nutrition for few calories.

HEALTH BENEFITS

Grapefruit is an excellent source of vitamin C. Pink and red grapefruit are good sources of disease-fighting beta-carotene. If you peel and eat a grapefruit like you would an orange, you get a good dose of cholesterol-lowering pectin from the membranes—the same soluble fiber that fills you up by dissolving in water and creating gels. As a member of the citrus family, grapefruit is also a storehouse of powerful phytochemicals such as flavonoids, terpenes, and limonoids. These naturally occurring substances may have cancer-preventing properties.

SELECTION AND STORAGE

Grapefruit isn't picked unless it's fully ripe, making selection a no-brainer. However, choose ones that are heavy for their size; they're juiciest. And avoid those that are soft or mushy, or oblong rather than round. They are generally of poorer quality—possibly pithy and less sweet.

GRAPEFRUIT, PINK OR RED
Serving Size: ½ fruit

Calories	37	Dietary Fiber	2 g
Fat	<1 g	Sodium	0 mg
Saturated Fat	0 g	Vitamin A	318 IU
Cholesterol	0 mg	Niacin	<1 mg
Carbohydrate	10 g	Vitamin C	47 mg
Protein	1 g	Potassium	158 mg

The difference in taste among white, red, and pink varieties of grapefruit is minimal; they are equally sweet (and equally tart). Store grapefruit in your refrigerator's crisper drawer; they'll keep for up to two months.

PREPARATION AND SERVING TIPS

Wash grapefruit before cutting to prevent bacteria that might be on the skin from being introduced to the inside. You might want to bring grapefruit to room temperature before you juice or slice it for better appreciation of flavor.

You don't have to relegate grapefruit to breakfast. Instead of halving and segmenting it, try peeling and eating it out of hand for a juicy, mouthwatering snack. For dessert, sprinkle with a little brown sugar and place it under the broiler until it bubbles.

GRAPES

Grapes, one of the oldest cultivated fruits, are unique because they grow on vines. This bite-size fruit is popular with everyone, especially kids (but be sure to peel or slice them lengthwise for young children to avoid choking). One of grapes' best attributes is that everyone likes them. Moreover, they're portable and neat, making them easy low-fat substitutes for high-fat, calorie-filled snacks and desserts. Bursting with juice, they are a refreshing way to fight the fat. You just have to be sure to have them handy.

HEALTH BENEFITS

Grapes may not be packed with traditional nutrients, but they do contain a collection of phytochemicals that researchers are just beginning to appreciate. Among them is ellagic acid, a natural substance also found in strawberries that is thought to possess cancer-preventing properties. Grapes also contain boron, a mineral believed to play a role in preventing the bone-destroying disease osteoporosis.

SELECTION AND STORAGE

Some varieties of grapes are available year-round. When buying grapes, look for clusters with plump, well-colored fruit attached to pliable, green stems. Soft or wrinkled grapes or those with bleached areas around the stem are past their prime.

There are basically three categories of grapes: the greens, the reds, and the blue/blacks. Good color is the key to good fla-

Grapes, American
Serving Size: 20 grapes

Calories 30	Dietary Fiber ....<1 g
Fat..............................<1 g	Sodium.......................0 mg
Saturated Fat.........0 g	Vitamin B$_6$ ....2 mg
Cholesterol.................0 mg	Manganese ....<1 mg
Carbohydrate ....8 g	Potassium ....92 mg
Protein ....<1 g	

vor. The sweetest green grapes are yellow-green in color; red varieties that are predominantly crimson/red will have the best flavor; and blue/black varieties taste best if their color is deep and rich, almost black. If you object to seeds, look for seedless varieties. Store grapes unwashed in the refrigerator. They'll keep up to a week.

Preparation and Serving Tips

Just before eating, rinse grape clusters and drain or pat dry. Slight chilling enhances the flavor and texture of table grapes. Cold, sliced grapes taste great blended in with low-fat yogurt. Frozen grapes make a popular summer treat. For a change of pace, skewer grapes, banana slices (dipped in lemon), apple chunks, and pineapple cubes, or any favorite fruit. Brush with a combination of honey, lemon, and ground nutmeg. Broil until warm.

GREENS FOR COOKING

Most often thought of as a Southern dish, collard greens and their cousins—beet greens, dandelion greens, mustard greens, and turnip greens—are gaining new respect as nutrition powerhouses—they're loaded with disease-fighting beta-carotene and offer respectable amounts of vitamin C, calcium, and fiber. All these attributes make cooking greens a wise choice for your diet. As fat-fighters, they play the part of most vegetables, providing little natural fat but filling stomachs with some fiber and furnishing nutrients galore. Just lose the traditional way of cooking them in bacon grease to turn them into true fat-fighting foods.

HEALTH BENEFITS

If you're keeping calories to a minimum, you depend on certain foods to provide more than their share of certain nutrients. And cooking greens fill that role for two nutrients in particular.

First, greens contribute an important nondairy source of calcium that's absorbed almost as well as the calcium found in dairy products. That's good news for those facing the threat of osteoporosis, as calcium is one of many factors crucial to bone health.

Second, most greens are superb sources of vitamin A, mostly in the form of beta-carotene, which has been shown to help protect against cancer, heart disease, and cataracts through its antioxidant properties. Other carotenoids found in greens may be just as potent cancer conquerors as well, but research is still lacking. The outer leaves of greens usually contain more beta-carotene than do the inner leaves. Dandelion greens are bursting with twice the vitamin A of other greens.

Some greens—collard, mustard, and turnip—belong to the cruciferous family, which also includes broccoli, cabbage, and cauliflower. Research has shown that people who eat a lot of cruciferous vegetables are less likely to suffer cancer than those whose diets contain fewer servings.

Some greens stand out individually. Beet greens shine in several minerals, including iron, as well as potassium, but they are also naturally high in sodium. Turnip greens provide folic acid—important for the prevention of birth defects and heart disease—plus manganese and copper. They are much richer in fiber and calcium than other greens.

SELECTION AND STORAGE

Choose greens that have smooth, green, firm leaves. Small, young leaves are likely to be the least bitter and most tender. Be sure the produce department kept the greens well-chilled, or they'll be bitter. Wilting is a sign of bitter-tasting greens.

COLLARD GREENS, COOKED
Serving Size: ½ cup

Calories 56	Dietary Fiber ....<1 g
Fat............................<1 g	Sodium.....................18 mg
Saturated Fat.........0 g	Vitamin A............2,109 IU
Cholesterol.................0 mg	Vitamin C ....9 mg
Carbohydrate ....3 g	Calcium....................74 mg
Protein........................1 g	

— Greens for Cooking

Unwashed greens store well for three to five days when wrapped in a damp paper towel and stored in an airtight plastic bag. The longer they are stored, however, the more bitter they will be. Be sure to wash greens well and remove the tough stems; cook only the leaves. One pound of raw leaves yields about a half cup of cooked greens.

Preparation and Serving Tips

Cook greens in a small amount of water, or steam them, to preserve their vitamin C content. Cook with the lid off to prevent the greens from turning a drab olive color. When you can, strain the nutritious cooking liquid and use it as a base for soups or stews.

Greens will overpower a salad. To eat them as a side dish, simmer in seasoned water or broth until wilted (collards may need to cook longer). Or you can combine greens with other vegetables and a whole grain for a healthful stir-fry dish. Finally, add them to soups and stews, where their strong flavor is an advantage.

Beet Greens, Cooked
Serving Size: ½ cup

Calories	20	Vitamin A	3,672 IU
Fat	<1 g	Vitamin C	18 mg
Saturated Fat	0 g	Riboflavin	<1 mg
Cholesterol	0 mg	Calcium	82 mg
Carbohydrate	4 g	Copper	<1 mg
Protein	2 g	Iron	1 mg
Dietary Fiber	1 g	Magnesium	49 mg
Sodium	173 mg	Potassium	654 mg

GREENS FOR SALADS

Everyone knows salads are diet food. Yet a heavy hand with dressing will do the healthiest salad in. Still, eaten before a meal, a salad can take the edge off hunger, while filling your stomach with its bulk. This should curb your appetite enough to modulate overindulgence for the rest of the meal. Though Romaine provides decent nutrition, most lettuce does not, so to make the ultimate fat-fighting salad, don't overlook greens. Wonderfully flavored greens like raddichio, arugula, endive, chicory, and escarole make a salad stand out in taste and nutrition. Some greens back up their fat-fighting bulk with a decent amount of fiber.

HEALTH BENEFITS

The darker the color of the salad green, the more nutritious it is. Beta-carotene is the chief disease-fighting nutrient found in the darker-colored greens. As an antioxidant, it battles certain cancers, heart disease, and cataracts. A dark-green color also indicates the presence of folic acid, which helps prevent neural-tube birth defects in the beginning stages of pregnancy. Researchers are uncovering other important contributions folic acid has to offer to your well-being like its role in the prevention of heart disease.

Chicory is a good source of vitamin C, another antioxidant nutrient linked to prevention of heart disease, cancer, and cataracts. Some salad greens, including arugula and watercress, are members of the cruciferous family, adding more ammunition to the fight against cancer.

— Greens for Salads

Selection and Storage

Avoid salad greens that are wilted or have brown-edged or slimy leaves. Once they reach this point, there's no bringing them back to life. They should have vivid color, and leaves should be firm. Store greens in your refrigerator's crisper drawer, roots intact, in perforated plastic bags.

Romaine is a produce-department staple, though it may never completely take the place of the boring, yet popular, iceberg. Less-recognizable greens come in a wider variety of sizes, shapes, and colors, and some manufacturers prepack a variety of these delicious treasures in handy salad packs.

Arugula: Also known as rocket or roquette, these small, flat leaves have a hot, peppery flavor. The older and larger the leaves, the more mustardlike the flavor. You're more likely to find arugula in ethnic or farmers' markets than in supermarkets. It's so delicate, it keeps for only a day or two.

Chicory: This curly-leaved green is sometimes mistakenly called curly endive. The dark-green leaves have a bitter taste but work well in salads with well-seasoned dressings.

Endive: Belgian endive and white chicory are names for this pale salad green. The small, cigar-shaped head has tightly packed leaves and a slightly bitter flavor. Endive stays fresh for three to four days.

Escarole: A close cousin to chicory, escarole is actually a type of endive. It has broad, slightly curved green leaves, with a milder flavor than Belgian endive.

Radicchio: Though it looks like a miniature head of red cabbage, this salad green is actually a member of the chicory family, with a less bitter flavor. Radicchio keeps up to a week.

ROMAINE LETTUCE
Serving Size: ½ cup, shredded

Calories......................4		Sodium......................2 mg	
Fat.............................<1 g		Calcium....................10 mg	
Saturated Fat.........0 g		Potassium ....81 mg	
Cholesterol.................0 mg		Vitamin A................728 IU	
Carbohydrate ....1 g		Folic Acid ....38 mcg	
Protein........................1 g		Vitamin C ....7 mg	
Dietary Fiber ....<1 g			

Romaine: Also known as cos, Romaine lettuce has long leaves that are crisp, with an oh-so-slight bitter taste. Romaine is hearty, storing well for up to ten days.

Watercress: This delicate green is sold in "bouquets," or trimmed and sealed in vacuum packs. Choose dark-green, glossy leaves and store in plastic bags; use in a day or two. Unopened vacuum packs last up to three days.

PREPARATION AND SERVING TIPS

Dirt and grit often settle between the leaves of salad greens. Separate the leaves, then wash well before using. For small bunches, swish leaves in a bowl of water.

In general, the stronger and more bitter the salad green, the stronger-flavored the dressing should be. Try warm mustard or garlic-based dressings with strong-flavored salad greens. But keep fat down: Rely more on vinegar than oil, or use low-fat yogurt or buttermilk as a base.

HERBS & SPICES

There are dozens upon dozens of herbs and spices, from commonplace black pepper to more exotic turmeric and cardamom. But all share two unique features—they add flavor and aroma to food, especially low-fat dishes where flavor can sometimes be lacking. Herbs and spices, then, are necessities in the fight against fat. Too often, they are relegated to attractively labeled bottles on revolving spice racks. This is unfortunate, because using the right blend of these taste enhancers can literally make or break a dish.

HEALTH BENEFITS

Most dried herbs and spices are low in calories, providing no more than 15 calories per teaspoon. So feel free to use them even if you are following a low-calorie regimen. Some are surprisingly good sources of nutrients. Paprika is an excellent source of vitamin A, parsley is rich in vitamin C, cumin is an unexpected source of iron, and caraway seeds even contribute a little calcium to your diet.

New research findings suggest that several herbs are also rich sources of antioxidants that may possibly prevent the growth of cancer cells and protect delicate arteries from buildup of cholesterol-filled plaque. Among them: allspice, basil, clove, coriander, dill, fennel leaves, mint, nutmeg, parsley, rosemary, and sage.

Aside from their nutrient and antioxidant contents, there are many health claims made for individual herbs. Here are but a few: Mint relieves gas and nausea; cinnamon enhances insulin's activity; oregano has antiseptic properties; sage contains compounds that act as antibiotics; thyme is said to relieve cramps. Most, however, have not been scientifically proved.

Selection and Storage

In our opinion, fresh is best. But it's not always easy to find fresh herbs. Farmers' markets are your best bet. Supermarkets may carry them sporadically, but often only in summer (although many supermarkets will special order them if you ask). You may find them through mail order catalogues, or you can grow your own windowsill herb garden. In any case, buy fresh herbs only as you need them. Wrap them in damp paper towels, place in a plastic bag, and refrigerate. They should last a few days.

When fresh aren't available, dried will do. Store dried herbs and spices in airtight containers, away from heat and light (over the stove is the worst spot). Dried herbs will keep for a year. Whole spices, like cloves or cinnamon, keep much longer. The flavor of dried herbs tends to fade faster than that of dried spices.

Preparation and Serving Tips

Becoming acquainted with herbs and spices is a must if you're committed to low-fat or low-salt cooking. When you remove fat or salt, a lot of flavor goes with it. That loss of flavor can be masked with herbs and spices.

If you're a novice at using herbs and spices, start by using only one or two per dish. If you're using fresh herbs, don't be shy. Their flavors are often subtle, and it usually takes more than you think to overpower a dish. With dried herbs, however, a little often goes a long way, so use judiciously. Start with

— Herbs & Spices

about ¼ to ⅓ teaspoon until you get a better "feel" for the amount you like in dishes.

If you're cooking with fresh herbs, wait until the end of the cooking time to add them, so they'll retain their delicate flavor. Dried herbs and spices, on the other hand, hold their flavor well—even under intense heat.

Here are some seasoning suggestions to get you started:

Pasta: basil, fennel, garlic, paprika, parsley, sage

Potatoes: chives, garlic, paprika, parsley, rosemary

Rice: cumin, marjoram, parsley, saffron, tarragon, thyme, turmeric

Salads: basil, chervil, chives, dillweed, marjoram, mint, parsley, tarragon

Seafood: chervil, dill, fennel, tarragon, parsley

Vegetables: basil, caraway, chives, dillweed, marjoram, mint, nutmeg, oregano, paprika, rosemary, savory, tarragon, thyme

KALE

Kale is king. Along with broccoli, it is one of the nutrition stand-outs among vegetables. It fights fat through its ability to mingle in a variety of roles—in side dishes, combined in main dishes, or in salads. For a green, kale is unusually high in fiber. This helps create the bulk you need to fill you up. It also pumps you up with nutrients, like calcium.

HEALTH BENEFITS

Though greens in general are nutritious foods, kale stands a head above the rest. Not only is it one of your best sources of beta-carotene, one of the antioxidants believed by many nutrition experts to be a major player in the battle against cancer, heart disease, and cataracts, it also provides other important nutrients.

According to recent research results, kale is an incredible source of well-absorbed calcium, which is one of the many factors that may help prevent osteoporosis. It also provides decent amounts of vitamin C, folic acid, magnesium, and potassium.

Don't forget, kale's a member of the cruciferous family, along with broccoli, brussels sprouts, cabbage, cauliflower, and collard greens. Many researchers believe that loading up on cruciferous vegetables can help ward off certain cancers.

SELECTION AND STORAGE

Kale looks like a darker green version of collards, but with frills. It also has a stronger flavor and a somewhat coarser tex-

Kale, Cooked

Serving Size: ½ cup

Calories	21	Sodium	15 mg
Fat	<1 g	Vitamin A	4,810 IU
Saturated Fat	0 g	Folic Acid	9 mcg
Cholesterol	0 mg	Vitamin C	27 mg
Carbohydrate	4 g	Calcium	47 mg
Protein	1 g	Magnesium	15 mg
Dietary Fiber	3 g	Potassium	148 mg

ture. The smaller leaves are more tender and the flavor is more mild, but it grows stronger the longer it is stored. So unless you actually prefer a strong taste, use kale within a day or two of buying it. Wrap fresh kale in damp paper towels, and store it in a plastic bag in the crisper drawer of your refrigerator.

PREPARATION AND SERVING TIPS

Wash kale thoroughly before cooking, as it often has dirt and sand in its leaves. Hearty kale stands up well to cooking, so just about any method will do. But keep cooking time to a minimum to preserve nutrients and to keep kale's strong odor from permeating the kitchen.

Simmer the greens in a well-seasoned stock for 10 to 30 minutes, until tender. Don't forget that most greens cook down a great deal. One pound of raw yields only about a half cup of cooked. Kale also works well in stir-fries, soups, and stews.

KIWIFRUIT

The funny-looking green fruit in the fuzzy brown package hit this country by storm a few years back. Now it's almost as commonplace as apples and bananas. Though native to China—as the "Chinese gooseberry"—a marketing campaign renamed this unusual fruit to one more suited to its new imported home—New Zealand. Today, it is grown in California. Kiwis carry a lot of nutrition in a small package. They aren't high in calories, yet they pack a powerful punch with their strong tart taste, which allows them to jazz up the flavor of low-fat diets.

HEALTH BENEFITS

Kiwifruit is literally filled with fiber. All those little black seeds combine for a good dose of insoluble fiber, which aids digestion by decreasing the transit time of stools through your system. But kiwifruit also offers soluble fiber, providing bulk that promotes the feeling of fullness—a natural diet aid. By creating gel-like substances that trap bile acids, it has the potential to reduce blood cholesterol levels.

Kiwis are brimming with vitamin C, which is essential for healthy gums and important for wound healing, and boasts ample amounts of good-for-your-bones magnesium and potassium.

SELECTION AND STORAGE

Because New Zealand and California have opposite seasons, and, therefore, opposite harvests, kiwis are available year-round. Choose those that are fairly firm, but give under slight pressure. Firm kiwis need about a week to ripen at room temperature. You can hasten the process by placing them in a closed paper bag. Store the bag at room temperature and begin checking for ripeness after two days. Ripe kiwis keep for one to two weeks in the refrigerator.

PREPARATION AND SERVING TIPS

With its brilliant green color and its inner circle of tiny black seeds, sliced kiwis are the perfect garnish. They don't even discolor when exposed to air since they contain so much vitamin C, which contains antioxidant properties that prevent oxygen from oxidizing the fruit and turning it brown.

Most people prefer eating peeled kiwifruit, though the skin is edible—just rub off the brown fuzz. You can slice kiwi, or peel it and eat it whole. Since kiwifruit contains a "tenderizing" enzyme that prevents gelatin from setting, it's a good idea to leave kiwifruit out of molded salads.

KIWIFRUIT
Serving Size: 1 medium

Calories	46	Dietary Fiber	3 g
Fat	<1 g	Sodium	4 mg
Saturated Fat	0 g	Vitamin C	75 mg
Cholesterol	0 mg	Calcium	20 mg
Carbohydrate	11 g	Magnesium	23 mg
Protein	1 g	Potassium	252 mg

LEMONS & LIMES

Probably the most tart of fruits, lemons and limes are rarely eaten alone. But their tart juice adds life to everything from salads to pies. This gives them *carte blanche* to fight fat by perking up the bland flavor of low-fat foods.

HEALTH BENEFITS

Anyone cutting back on fat or salt should keep a lemon or lime handy. Squeeze on lemon or lime juice, add a few herbs, and you can perk up most any dish. Neither juice adds any appreciable calories, just pizzazz, plus a bit of nutrition, too.

Both lemons and limes exude vitamin C, the antioxidant that helps fight heart disease and cancer. Moreover, lemons and limes contain phytochemicals, such as terpenes and limonenes, that may play a role in preventing some cancers.

SELECTION AND STORAGE

Look for firm, unblemished fruit that's heavy for its size—an indicator of juiciness. Thin-skinned fruit yields the most juice. Refrigerated, they keep for a month or two. Lemons will even keep for a week or two at room temperature, but limes must be refrigerated.

Lemon varieties vary mostly in their skin thickness, juiciness, and number of seeds. The key lime—of pie fame—is more flavorful than other lime varieties because of its greater acidity. Key limes are small and round; other varieties look more like green lemons. Limes typically turn yellowish as they ripen. The greenest limes have the best flavor.

LIME
Serving Size: 1 medium

Calories 20	Dietary Fiber ....2 g
Fat............................<1 g	Sodium.......................1 mg
Saturated Fat.........0 g	Folic Acid ....6 mcg
Cholesterol.................0 mg	Vitamin C ....20 mg
Carbohydrate ....7 g	Calcium.....................22 mg
Protein ....<1 g	Potassium ....68 mg

LEMON
Serving Size: 1 medium

Calories 17	Dietary Fiber ....3 g
Fat............................<1 g	Sodium.......................1 mg
Saturated Fat.........0 g	Folic Acid ....6 mcg
Cholesterol.................0 mg	Vitamin C ....31 mg
Carbohydrate .... 5 g	Calcium.....................15 mg
Protein ....<1 g	Potassium ....80 mg

PREPARATION AND SERVING TIPS

To get more juice from a lemon or lime, bring it to room temperature, then roll it back and forth under the palm of your hand before you cut and squeeze it.

The most flavorful part of the fruit is its "zest," or skin. Scrape it off with a grater or knife and use it to enhance desserts and fruit salads.

A twist of lemon also adds zing to fish.

LENTILS

Because they boast a bevy of low-fat nutrients, lentils are finally gaining the recognition they deserve as a great source of low-fat protein, making them the perfect substitute for meat.

HEALTH BENEFITS

Lentils' high fiber content is a boon to health; it's mostly the soluble kind, so it lowers blood cholesterol by creating gels that bind with bile acids, forcing the body to use cholesterol to replace them. These gels also tie up carbohydrates, so they are absorbed more slowly, keeping you full longer—of benefit to anyone on a diet.

Lentils are exceptionally high in folic acid, which can help prevent certain birth defects and may prevent heart disease as well. Lentils are an important source of iron for vegetarians, serving as protection against anemia.

SELECTION AND STORAGE

Brown, green, and red lentils are the most common varieties in the United States. Most supermarkets carry them packaged, but you can buy them in bulk at health-food stores and gourmet markets.

If you buy them packaged, look for well-sealed containers, with uniformly sized, brightly colored, disk-shaped lentils. If you buy them in bulk, check the lentils for tiny pinholes. Don't buy them if you spot holes; they're a sign of insect infestation.

When stored in a well-sealed container at a cool temperature, lentils keep for up to a year.

PREPARATION AND SERVING TIPS

Red lentils cook quickly and become mushy, so they work best in dishes where a firm texture isn't a concern, like in soups, purees, or dips. Brown or green lentils, on the other hand, retain their shape if not overcooked and can be used in salads or any dish in which you don't want your lentils reduced to mush.

Most lentils cook in 30 to 45 minutes or less and they don't require any precooking soak like dried beans do.

Best of all, lentils are willing recipients of flavorful herbs and spices, taking on the flavors of the foods they are mixed with. No wonder they are common in Indian, Middle Eastern, and African recipes.

LENTILS

Serving Size: ½ cup, cooked

Calories	115	Thiamin	<1 mg
Fat	<1 g	Vitamin B6	<1 mg
Saturated Fat	<1 g	Calcium	19 mg
Cholesterol	0 mg	Copper	<1 mg
Carbohydrate	20 g	Iron	3 mg
Protein	9 g	Magnesium	35 mg
Dietary Fiber	5 g	Manganese	<1 mg
Sodium	2 mg	Phosphorus	178 mg
Folic Acid	179 mcg	Potassium	366 mg
Niacin	1 mg	Zinc	1 mg

MANGOES

This "fruit of India," as it is sometimes called, is unique in its wealth of nutrients and richness of flavor. Though the pungent flavor may be an acquired taste for some, the one-two nutrition punch it delivers is worth it.

HEALTH BENEFITS

If you're limiting your intake of fat and calories, eating concentrated sources of nutrients makes sense. And mangoes deliver. Mangoes are a superior source of beta-carotene. In fact, they are one of the top beta-carotene providers you can eat. Consuming large amounts of this antioxidant has been linked to a reduced risk of some forms of cancers, including lung cancer.

Just one mango provides almost an entire day's worth of vitamin C. Unlike many other fruits, mangoes contribute several B vitamins and the minerals calcium and magnesium.

SELECTION AND STORAGE

There are hundreds of varieties of mangoes in every shape, size, and color. The color of mangoes ranges from yellow to red and will deepen as the fruit ripens, though some green may remain even in perfectly ripened fruits. When ripe, a mango has a sweet, perfumey smell. If it has a fermented aroma, then it's past its prime.

Choose mangoes that feel firm, but yield to slight pressure. The skin should be unbroken, and the color should have begun to change from green to yellow, orange, or red. Though

MANGOES
Serving Size: 1 mango

Calories	135	Niacin	1 mg
Fat	1 g	Riboflavin	<1 mg
Saturated Fat	<1 g	Thiamin	<1 mg
Cholesterol	0 mg	Vitamin B6	<1 mg
Carbohydrate	35 g	Vitamin C	57 mg
Protein	1 g	Calcium	21 mg
Dietary Fiber	6 g	Magnesium	18 mg
Sodium	4 mg	Potassium	322 mg
Vitamin A	8,060 IU		

it's normal for mangoes to have some black spots, avoid those mottled with too many. It's a sign the fruit is overripe. Ditto for loose or shriveled skin.

If you bring home a mango that isn't ripe, you can speed the process by placing it in a paper bag with a ripe mango. Check daily to avoid overripening.

PREPARATION AND SERVING TIPS

Because mangoes are so juicy, they can be a real mess to cut and serve. You can peel the fruit and eat it as you would a peach, just be sure to have plenty of napkins or paper towels on hand to sop up the juice that runs down your chin.

Try eating chilled mangoes as dessert or as breakfast fruit. For extra zip, sprinkle them with a little lime juice. Mangoes are an indispensable ingredient in sauces and chutneys.

MELONS

Melons may come in different shapes, sizes, and colors, but they all have two things in common: a soft, sweet, juicy pulp and superb, natural low-fat taste—that's why it's hard to say no to melons. Besides being low in fat, melons offer a decent dose of fiber, which helps fill you up. As a snack for dieters, melons can't be beat. Their juicy sweetness is just the substitute for fat-filled snacks and desserts.

HEALTH BENEFITS

Most melons are rich in potassium, a nutrient that may help control blood pressure and possibly prevent strokes. They're also abundant in vitamin C, one arm of the now-famous disease-fighting antioxidant trio. Another arm that's well represented is beta-carotene. Researchers believe that beta-carotene and vitamin C are capable of preventing heart disease, cancer, and other chronic conditions. No matter which way you cut them, when it comes to nutrition, melons are number one.

SELECTION AND STORAGE

The three most popular melons in the United States are cantaloupe, watermelon, and honeydew. In general, look for melons that are evenly shaped with no bruises, cracks, or soft spots. Select melons that are heavy for their size; they tend to be juicier.

Cantaloupes should have a prominent light brown netting that stands out from the underlying smooth skin. If the stem is still attached, the melon was picked too early. Ripe can-taloupes have a mildly sweet fragrance. If the cantaloupe smells sickeningly sweet, or if there is mold where the stem used to be, it is probably overripe and quite possibly rotten. Cantaloupes continue to ripen off the vine, so if you buy it ripe, eat it as soon as possible.

Choosing a watermelon is a little chancier. Watermelons don't ripen much after they are picked, so what you see is what you get. The single most reliable sign of ripeness is a firm underside with a yellowish color; if it is white or green, the melon is not yet mature. A whole watermelon keeps in the refrigerator up to a week, but cut watermelon should be eaten as soon as possible. The flesh deteriorates rapidly, taking on an unappetizing slimy texture.

Ripe honeydew, signaled by a yellowish-white color, are the sweetest of the melons. Avoid those that are paper-white or greenish white; they'll never ripen. If the skin of a honeydew is smooth, it was picked prematurely. It should have a slightly

CANTALOUPE
Serving Size: ½ melon

Calories	94	Vitamin A	8,608 IU
Fat	1 g	Folic Acid	46 mcg
Saturated Fat	na	Niacin	2 mg
Cholesterol	0 mg	Vitamin B_6	<1 mg
Carbohydrate	22 g	Vitamin C	113 mg
Protein	2 g	Calcium	28 mg
Dietary Fiber	3 g	Magnesium	28 mg
Sodium	23 mg	Potassium	825 mg

WATERMELON
Serving Size: ¹⁄₁₆ fruit

Calories	152	Niacin	1 mg
Fat	2 g	Pantothenic Acid	1 mg
Saturated Fat	na	Thiamin	<1 mg
Cholesterol	0 mg	Vitamin B₆	1 mg
Carbohydrate	35 g	Vitamin C	47 mg
Protein	3 g	Calcium	38 mg
Dietary Fiber	3 g	Magnesium	52 mg
Sodium	10 mg	Potassium	560 mg
Vitamin A	1,762 IU	Copper	2 mg

wrinkled feel. Honeydews keep longer than cantaloupes, but should still be refrigerated. Try to cut it open within four to five days. When you do, leave the seeds in place until you're ready to eat it; they help keep the fruit moist.

PREPARATION AND SERVING TIPS

Some people like melons only slightly chilled or even room temperature, but watermelons taste best when they're served icy cold. A multicolored melon-ball salad topped with fresh, chopped mint makes a pretty dessert. Chilled melon soup is a refreshing change of pace in hot weather. And the natural cavity left in a cantaloupe after removing the seeds is a perfect place for fillers like nonfat yogurt or fruit salad.

MILK, SKIM

Milk is nicknamed "nature's most perfect food." While it's not truly perfect, skim milk certainly comes close with its high protein and exceptional calcium counts and a bevy of B vitamins. All this for only 86 calories in an eight-ounce glass. In fact, merely switching from whole milk to skim milk can be one of the more significant choices you can make to reduce fat and calories in your diet.

Though milk is often thought of as highly allergenic, only a tiny fraction of people are truly allergic to milk. Gastrointestinal distress after drinking milk is more likely the result of lactose intolerance, a much more common problem. A large percentage of the world's population—though far fewer in the United States—suffer from lactose intolerance, the inability to digest lactose, the natural sugar in milk. New research, however, claims gastrointestinal symptoms are often incorrectly attributed to this condition. Even those in the study who proved to be lactose intolerant were able to enjoy at least a cup of milk a day without experiencing digestive distress.

HEALTH BENEFITS

The advantage of skim milk over whole milk cannot be stressed enough. The fat in whole milk is mostly saturated animal fat—the kind that raises blood cholesterol. And when you compare the percentage of calories from fat per serving, whole milk checks in at 50 percent; skim milk at 4 percent. So you can really see the fat savings you'll reap if you make the switch. And if you do it gradually, switching first to 2 percent, then 1 percent, then skim, the transition is painless.

MILK, SKIM

Serving Size: 8 oz

Calories	86	Vitamin B$_{12}$	1 mcg
Fat	<1 g	Niacin	<1 mg
Saturated Fat	<1 g	Pantothenic Acid	1 mg
Cholesterol	4 mg	Riboflavin	<1 mg
Carbohydrate	12 g	Vitamin D	3 mcg
Protein	8 g	Calcium	302 mg
Dietary Fiber	0 g	Phosphorus	247 mg
Sodium	126 mg	Potassium	406 mg
Vitamin A	500 IU		

Switching to skim milk won't compromise the amount of nutrients in your glass. If anything, you'll get slightly more. Fat takes up a lot of space, leaving less room for nutrients, so when the fat content is decreased, there's more room for nutrients. Skim milk is an excellent source of calcium, which plays a critical role in preventing osteoporosis. And the calcium in milk may be better absorbed than the calcium found in supplements, because lactose, which is also found in milk, but not in supplements, appears to aid its absorption.

Milk in this country is fortified with vitamins A and D and is the major dietary source of both. It's also one of the major contributors of riboflavin, a B vitamin involved in the breakdown of food.

SELECTION AND STORAGE

All milk should have a sell-by date stamped on the carton. Don't depend on milk to stay fresh much longer than the date on the carton.

– Milk, Skim

Milk in translucent plastic jugs is susceptible to considerable losses of riboflavin and vitamin A, much more so than milk in paper cartons. That's because light, even the fluorescent light in supermarkets, destroys these two light-sensitive nutrients. This same light also affects the taste of milk.

Whatever you do, don't buy raw milk or products made from raw milk, such as some cheeses. Raw milk has not been pasteurized and often carries bacteria that can make you sick. It's especially dangerous to give it to children, the elderly, or people with an impaired immune system.

PREPARATION AND SERVING TIPS

Milk tastes best when it's served icy cold. There are, of course, some recipes that just won't work well with skim milk, but most do fine. A tip: When you heat milk, don't allow it to come to a boil. This forms a film on the surface that won't dissolve.

MILLET

In the United States, millet is used mainly for fodder and bird-seed, but this nutritious grain is a staple in the diets of a large portion of the world's population, including Africa and Asia. It has been cultivated for about 6,000 years. There are several varieties of millet available throughout the world. In Ethiopia, it is used to make porridge; in India, to make roti (a traditional bread); and in the Caribbean, it is cooked with peas and beans.

HEALTH BENEFITS

Millet is a remarkable source of protein, making it perfect for vegetarian diets. It's also a good source of niacin, copper, and manganese. You may want to give millet a try if you are allergic to wheat. Chances are, you won't suffer a reaction.

SELECTION AND STORAGE

Look for this slightly bland-flavored grain in health food stores, Asian markets, and gourmet shops. Millet is a tiny, pale-yellow bead. Store it in an airtight container in a cool, dry place, and it should keep for up to a month. In the freezer it will keep up to a year.

You may occasionally see cracked millet sold as couscous. But couscous is most often made from semolina.

PREPARATION AND SERVING TIPS

Millet has no characteristic flavor of its own, and it tends to take on the flavor of the foods it is prepared with. To cook millet, add one cup of whole millet and a teaspoon of margarine or oil to two cups of boiling water. Simmer, covered for 25 to 30 minutes. It should double in volume, once all the water is absorbed. Keep it covered and undisturbed while it cooks, and you'll produce a millet that is fluffy; stir it often and it will have a creamy consistency, like a cooked cereal.

For a change from the same old thing, try millet on its own as a hot breakfast cereal. You can cook it with apple juice, instead of water, and top it off with raisins, brown sugar, or nuts.

Cooked millet can also be combined with cooked beans or peas to make vegetarian "burgers." Simply combine the two (they should be moist enough to hold together), and shape into patties.

Millet also works well in soups and stews. Simply rinse the millet in a strainer or colander and add to the mix. It should take about 20 to 30 minutes for the millet to absorb the liquid and become tender.

Millet

Serving Size: ½ cup

Calories...............143	Dietary Fiber...........4.3 g
Protein...................4.2 g	Sodium......................2 mg
Carbohydrate.........28.4 g	Niacin.....................1.6 mg
Fat..........................1.2 g	Copper....................0.2 mg
Saturated............0.2 g	Magnesium..............52 mg
Cholesterol...............0 mg	Manganese.............0.3 mg

MUSHROOMS

Mushrooms may be standard fare in Asian cultures, but Americans are only beginning to appreciate them for their ability to perk up low-fat dishes. Though low in fat, they contain a super-powerful flavor enhancer, glutamic acid, which is the same amino acid (a building block of protein) found in MSG (monosodium glutamate), except the mushroom variety isn't loaded with salt. Besides lending wonderful flavor to foods, mushrooms contribute more nutrition than you might think.

HEALTH BENEFITS

Mushrooms provide an unusual array of nutrients, not unlike those in meat, making them a particularly appropriate food for vegetarians. Cooked mushrooms are an unexpected protein source, which, even though incomplete, is easily complemented by grains. They also shine in iron, riboflavin, and niacin; offer decent amounts of potassium and zinc; and are full of fiber.

When possible, stick to cooked mushrooms. They're higher in nutrients than raw mushrooms; for the same volume, you get two, three, or even four times the nutrients. That's because cooking removes water from mushrooms, concentrating nutrients and flavor. Moreover, hydrazines—toxic natural compounds in raw mushrooms—are eliminated when mushrooms are cooked or dried.

Some researchers have found that cooked enoki, oyster, shiitake, pine, and straw mushrooms have antitumor activity.

BUTTON MUSHROOMS, FRESH, COOKED
Serving Size: ½ cup pieces

Calories	21	Sodium	2 mg
Fat	<1 g	Riboflavin	<1 mg
Saturated Fat	0 g	Niacin	4 mg
Cholesterol	0 mg	Iron	1 mg
Carbohydrate	4 g	Potassium	277 mg
Protein	2 g	Zinc	1 mg
Dietary Fiber	2 g		

Wood-ear mushrooms exhibit blood-thinning properties that may help prevent the dangerous clotting that contributes to heart disease.

SELECTION AND STORAGE

All supermarkets stock the white button mushroom, and many have expanded their selection to include the popular shiitake; trumpet-shaped chanterelle; sprout-like enoki; small, brown, intensely-flavored, spongy-capped morel; huge oyster; hearty-flavored portobello; and crunchy, often dried, Chinese wood-ear.

When selecting button mushrooms, look for those with caps that extend completely down to the stems, with no brown "gills" showing. If mushrooms have "opened"—meaning the gills are showing—they are older and won't last as long. They are perfectly acceptable to use, but they'll have a stronger flavor. The color should be creamy white or soft tan. Avoid those that have dark-brown soft spots or long, woody stems. Growers used to add sulfites to the packages to maintain their white color for longer periods of time, but this practice was discontinued—good news for those who are allergic to these additives.

Mushrooms like cool, humid, circulating air. So store them in a paper bag or ventilated container in your refrigerator, but not in the crisper drawer. Do not store them in a plastic bag; otherwise they'll get slimy. Mushrooms only last a couple of days, but you can still use them for flavoring even after they've turned brown.

A caution: Picking wild mushrooms can be hazardous to your health. There are too many poisonous varieties that fool even the most experienced foragers. So play it safe and stick to cultivated varieties of wild mushrooms.

PREPARATION AND SERVING TIPS

Don't wash mushrooms; they absorb water like a sponge. Use a mushroom brush or wipe with a barely damp cloth. Don't cut mushrooms until you're ready to use them; they'll darken. Use the trimmed stems to flavor soups.

Mushrooms cook quickly. Overcooking makes them rubbery and tough. If you sauté, go easy on the butter or margarine; they'll absorb it like water and you'll suffer the consequences. Try cooking them in a bit of wine instead. Due to their high water content, mushrooms add liquid to a dish once they cook down.

Nuts & Seeds

This category is just a little nutty. Besides seeds, it encompasses some foods that aren't true nuts but have similar nutrition. This includes peanuts (really legumes) and Brazil nuts and cashews, which are technically seeds. Because almost all nuts and seeds are super high in fat, it may surprise you that we are calling them fat-fighting foods. But the fat is unsaturated and may have disease-fighting properties. As long as you can restrain yourself, nuts and seeds can indeed be fat-fighters. By taking the place of more traditional protein sources, nuts and seeds can actually reduce the fat in your overall diet.

HEALTH BENEFITS

Nuts and seeds are good news/bad news foods. They are high in protein and nutrients, though their fat content—75 to 95 percent of total calories—precludes eating too many at a time. Macadamia, the gourmet of nuts, is the worst culprit. Chestnuts are the only truly low-fat nuts—only eight percent of their calories comes from fat.

Of all the nuts, peanuts provide the most complete protein. Other nuts are missing the amino acid lysine. But all are easily complemented by grains. As an alternative protein source, then, their fat content can be forgiven.

Recent research has heartened nut lovers. Studies at Loma Linda University in California found that eating nuts five times a week—about two ounces a day—lowered participants' blood cholesterol levels by 12 percent. Walnuts were used, but similar results have been reported with almonds and peanuts. The researchers theorize that replacing saturated fat in the diet with the monounsaturated fat in nuts may be the key. It makes sense, then, to eat nuts instead of other fatty foods, not just to gobble them down on top of your regular fare.

Some nuts, notably walnuts, are rich in omega-3 fatty acids, which may contribute further to the fight against heart disease and possibly even arthritis. Also, seeds and some nuts contain significant amounts of vitamin E. As an antioxidant, vitamin E can help prevent the oxidation of LDL cholesterol, which can damage arteries. More heartening news: Seeds are a good source of folic acid. Researchers have found that folic acid helps prevent the buildup of homocysteine. High levels of this amino acid have been linked to heart disease.

Seeds, peanuts, and peanut butter are super sources of niacin. Nuts are chock-full of hard-to-get minerals, such as copper, iron, and zinc. Seeds are among the better plant sources of iron and zinc. And nuts do their part to keep bones strong by providing magnesium, manganese, and boron.

PEANUT BUTTER, SMOOTH STYLE
Serving Size: 2 Tbsp

Calories	188	Niacin	4 mg
Fat	16 g	Vitamin E	3 mg
Saturated Fat	3 g	Copper	<1 mg
Cholesterol	0 mg	Magnesium	50 mg
Carbohydrate	7 g	Manganese	1 mg
Protein	8 g	Phosphorus	103 mg
Dietary Fiber	2 g	Potassium	231 mg
Sodium	153 mg	Zinc	1 mg

One caution: Brazil nuts are astonishingly high in selenium—perhaps too high. True, selenium is a beneficial antioxidant, but too much selenium is toxic. Stick to only one or two for a snack.

SELECTION AND STORAGE

Fresh nuts are available in fall and winter. Seeds and shelled nuts are available year-round, but check for a freshness date. If you buy bulk, they should smell fresh, not rancid. Aflatoxin, a known carcinogen produced by a mold that grows naturally on peanuts, can be a problem, so discard those that are discolored, shriveled, moldy, or taste bad. And stick to commercial brands of peanut butter. A survey found that best-selling brands contained only trace amounts of aflatoxin, supermarket brands had five times as much, while fresh-ground peanut butters averaged more than ten times as much.

Because of their high fat content, you must protect nuts from rancidity. Unshelled nuts can keep for a few months in a cool,

---

CASHEWS, DRY-ROASTED
Serving Size: 1 oz

Calories	163	Sodium	4 mg
Fat	13 g	Copper	1 mg
Saturated Fat	3 g	Iron	2 mg
Cholesterol	0 mg	Magnesium	74 mg
Carbohydrate	9 g	Phosphorus	139 mg
Protein	4 g	Zinc	2 mg
Dietary Fiber	2 g		

Sunflower Seed Kernels
Serving Size: 1 oz, oil-roasted

Calories	176	Niacin	1 mg
Fat	16 g	Vitamin E	14 mg
Saturated Fat	2 g	Copper	1 mg
Cholesterol	0 mg	Iron	2 mg
Carbohydrate	4 g	Magnesium	36 mg
Protein	6 g	Manganese	1 mg
Dietary Fiber	2 g	Phosphorus	323 mg
Sodium	1 mg	Zinc	2 mg
Folic Acid	67 mcg		

dry location. But once they're shelled or the container is opened, refrigerate or freeze them. Seeds with the hulls intact keep for several months if cool and dry; seed kernels don't keep as long.

PREPARATION AND SERVING TIPS

By using nuts in cooking and baking, you can benefit from their nutrition without overdoing fat and calories, since a little flavor goes a long way. Nuts on cereal can boost your morning fiber intake. Peanut butter on apple wedges or a slice of hearty whole-wheat toast is a superb breakfast or lunch.

A sprinkling of seed kernels over pasta, salads, and stir-fries adds crunch and flavor.

Tips: Brazil nuts open easier if chilled first; almonds should be boiled and then dunked in cold water to make peeling them a snap.

OATS

Whether horse feed or muffins come to mind when you think of oats, you're probably underestimating this truly healthful grain. Although its fat-fighting fiber has been sometimes maligned, rest assured it packs plenty of punch.

HEALTH BENEFITS

In the past few years, oat bran has risen and fallen from wonder-food status. While the media attention has vanished, oats remain as nutritious as ever, with the same fat-fighting potential for reducing the risk of disease as before.

A recent analysis of ten studies highlighted the effect of oats' soluble fiber—the same beta-glucans found in barley—on blood-cholesterol levels. On average, eating three grams of soluble (not total) fiber a day—the amount in two bowls of oatmeal or one cup of cooked oat bran—reduced cholesterol by six points in three months. Participants with the highest cholesterol levels saw the best response; those whose blood-cholesterol levels were over 230 mg/dL saw their levels drop by 16 points. Those who ate the most oat bran benefited the most. Another study showed that in certain individuals, oat bran can be as effective as—and certainly much less expensive than—medication in curbing elevated blood-cholesterol levels.

Similarly exciting results have been seen in people with diabetes and those with high-normal blood-sugar levels. The soluble fiber in oats means slower digestion, spreading the rise in blood sugar over a longer time period. Some people with diabetes who followed a diet high in soluble fiber from sources like oats and beans have been able to reduce their medication. Weight watchers benefit, too. The soluble fiber in oats fills you up by creating gels. The gels delay stomach emptying, so you feel full longer.

Oats have more to offer everyone. They are tops in protein and manganese—providing 50 percent of the recommended intake for this mineral. In addition, they offer an unusual amount of iron, thiamin, and magnesium.

Selection and Storage

The bran of the oat grain is the outer layer of the oat kernel, where much of the fiber and many of the nutrients reside. Whole oats—rolled or steel-cut—contain the bran along with the rest of the oat kernel. Oat bran contains the same nutrients and fiber found in whole oats but they are more concentrated. So eating whole oats will give you the same benefits of oat bran, you'll just need to eat more of it to get the same effect.

Cooking time and texture are the only differences among the varieties. Steel-cut oats, sometimes called Scotch oats or Irish oats, are whole oats sliced into long pieces. They have a chewy texture and take about 20 minutes to cook.

Rolled oats are steamed and flattened between steel rollers, so they take about five minutes to cook and are easier to chew than steel-cut oats.

Quick oats are cut into smaller pieces before being rolled, so they cook very quickly—in about a minute. But the time saved from cooking quick oats rather than rolled oats may not be worth it, considering what you sacrifice in flavor and texture.

Instant oats are precooked and pressed so thin it takes only boiling water to "reconstitute" them. Generally, they have a lot of added sodium; the flavored versions also have added sugar.

Store oats in a dark, dry location in a well-sealed container. Oats will keep up to a year. Whole oats are more likely to go rancid, so be sure to refrigerate them.

PREPARATION AND SERVING TIPS

To make oatmeal, all you do is simmer rolled oats in water on the stove for five minutes (one minute for quick oats). Do not overcook your oatmeal or you'll have a thick, gummy mess. If you like, sprinkle with cinnamon and top with skim milk. You couldn't find a more satisfying, low-fat, high-fiber way to start the day. Oat bran can be served as a hot cereal, too—it takes about six minutes to cook—though the taste might take some getting used to.

ROLLED OATS, COOKED (OATMEAL)
Serving Size: ¾ cup (⅓ cup uncooked)

Calories	108	Sodium	1 mg
Fat	2 g	Thiamin	<1 mg
Saturated Fat	<1 g	Iron	1 mg
Cholesterol	0 mg	Magnesium	42 mg
Carbohydrate	19 g	Manganese	1 mg
Protein	5 g	Phosphorus	133 mg
Dietary Fiber	3 g	Zinc	1 mg

Granola is traditionally made with oats. By making it yourself, you can avoid the fat trap that many commercial varieties fall into. First, toast the oats in a shallow pan in an oven preheated to 300°F, stirring occasionally until brown. Then combine the oats with wheat germ, raisins, your favorite nuts or seeds (toasted), dried fruit if you like, and a little honey. Let the mixture cool, then store it in an air-tight container in the refrigerator.

Whole oats can be cooked (simmer for six minutes) and combined with rice for a pilaf, or mixed with vegetables and seeds for a main dish.

Both oat bran and oats (rolled or quick) can be used in baking. Oats alone don't contain enough gluten to make bread, but you can modify your recipes to include half the grain as oats.

ONIONS

The onion is a member of the allium family, which, as your nose will tell you, also includes garlic, shallots, leeks, and chives. Egyptians worshiped the onion's many layers as a symbol of eternity. Today, the onion can be one of the most useful and flavorful ingredients in creating low-fat, healthful dishes.

HEALTH BENEFITS

While dry onions are a surprising source of fiber, they are not particularly rich in any other nutrients. Green onions, on the other hand, have those green tops, which provide a wealth of vitamin A. Without their flavor, some low-fat foods would be far too bland for most of us.

Moreover, like garlic, onions are just now being appreciated for their contributions to health. Research has lagged behind that of garlic, but there are promising signs that onions have similar anticancer and cholesterol-lowering properties. Onions may also play a role in preventing blood clots and alleviating the symptoms of allergies and asthma.

SELECTION AND STORAGE

Dry onions are any common onion—yellow, white, or red—that does not require refrigeration. This distinguishes them from green onions, which will perish quickly when stored at room temperature.

Dry onions come in various shapes and colors, none of which is a reliable indicator of taste or strength. The white, or yellow globe, onion keeps its pungent flavor when cooked. All-purpose white or yellow onions are milder. Sweet onions—Bermuda, Spanish, and Italian—are the mildest.

Choose firm dry onions with shiny, tissue-thin skins. "Necks" should be tight and dry. If they look too dry or discolored or have soft, wet spots, don't buy them—they aren't fresh.

Dry onions keep three to four weeks if stored in a dry, dark, cool location. Don't store them next to potatoes, which give off a gas that'll cause onions to decay. Light turns onions bitter. A cut onion should be wrapped in plastic, refrigerated, and used within a day or two.

Green onions, also called "spring" onions because that's the time of the year when they are harvested, have small white bulbs and are topped by thin green stalks. Though they are often sold as scallions, true scallions are just straight green stalks with no bulb. Look for green onions with crisp, not wilted, tops. For pungent aroma, choose fatter bulbs; for a sweeter taste, smaller bulbs are your best bet.

Green onions must be refrigerated. They keep best in a plastic bag in your refrigerator's crisper drawer.

ONION, DRY
Serving Size: ½ cup chopped

Calories 29	Protein........................1 g
Fat............................<1 g	Dietary Fiber ....2 g
Cholesterol.................0 mg	Sodium......................8 mg
Saturated Fat.........0 g	Vitamin C ....6 mg
Carbohydrate ....7 g	Vitamin B$_6$ ....<1 mg

PREPARATION AND SERVING TIPS

To keep tears from flowing, try slicing onions under running water. Or chill onions for an hour before cutting. To get the onion smell off your hands, rub your fingers with lemon juice or vinegar.

Onions are the perfect seasoning for almost any cooked dish. Their flavor mellows when they are cooked because smelly sulfur compounds are converted to sugar when heated. Onions sauté wonderfully, even without butter. Use a non-stick skillet and perhaps a teaspoon of olive oil. Keep heat low or they'll scorch and turn bitter.

Sweet onions are ideal raw, as rings in salads or as slices atop sandwiches. They add bite to a three-bean salad or a plate of homegrown tomatoes.

Wash green onions, trimming roots and dry leaves. Chop up bulb, stalk, and all. They work well in stir-fry dishes, adding an understated bite. Green onions can also be served raw with low-fat dip as part of a crudités platter.

GREEN ONION, FRESH
Serving Size: ½ cup chopped (stalks and bulbs)

Calories	13	Dietary Fiber	1 g
Fat	<1 g	Sodium	2 mg
Saturated Fat	0 g	Vitamin A	2,500 IU
Cholesterol	0 mg	Vitamin C	23 mg
Carbohydrate	3 g	Iron	1 mg
Protein	1 g		

Oranges & Tangerines

Oranges and tangerines are staples of American diets, and fortunately, they fit nicely into a fat-fighting diet; they are sweet enough to satisfy as snacks and desserts, making them wonderful substitutes for fat-filled sweets.

HEALTH BENEFITS

Oranges are most famous, of course, for their vitamin C. One orange provides 134 percent of the RDA. That's particularly important for smokers, who may require twice as much vitamin C as nonsmokers to help ward off the development of lung cancer. For women in their childbearing years, oranges are a great source of folic acid, now known to help prevent neural-tube birth defects.

Tangerines only have a third as much vitamin C and folic acid as oranges, but they provide three times as much cancer-fighting vitamin A.

SELECTION AND STORAGE

Oranges are one of the few fruits abundant in winter. There are more than 100 varieties in all, but your supermarket probably carries only a few.

The California navels, with their telltale "belly-buttons," easy-to-peel thick skins, and easy-to-segment flesh with no annoying seeds, are the favorite eating oranges. The Valencias, pride of Florida, are the premier juice oranges. Mandarin oranges are small and sweet with thin skins and easily sectioned segments. Tangerines are a popular type of mandarin.

NAVEL ORANGE, FRESH
Serving Size: 1 small

Calories 65	Dietary Fiber ....2 g
Fat...............................<1 g	Sodium........................1 mg
Saturated Fat.........0 g	Vitamin C ....80 mg
Cholesterol..................0 mg	Folic Acid ....47 mcg
Carbohydrate ....16 g	Calcium.....................56 mg
Protein........................1 g	Potassium ....250 mg

TANGERINE, FRESH
Serving Size: 1 medium

Calories 37	Protein........................1 g
Fat...............................<1 g	Dietary Fiber ....2 g
Saturated Fat.........0 g	Sodium........................1 mg
Cholesterol..................0 mg	Vitamin A................773 IU
Carbohydrate ....9 g	Vitamin C ....26 mg

For all varieties, select firm fruit heavy for its size, indicating juiciness. Green color and blemishes are fine. Refrigerated, most varieties, except mandarins, will keep for two weeks.

PREPARATION AND SERVING TIPS

For fruit salads, choose seedless oranges or tangerines, such as navels or canned mandarins. Use orange juice to make marinades or nonfat sauces. Or blend with a banana and skim milk for a delicious, low-fat shake.

PARSNIPS

Parsnips look like anemic carrots, certainly not as appealing as you'd think, given their medieval reputation as an aphrodisiac. But they're nutritious just the same.

HEALTH BENEFITS

Parsnips shine as a fiber source. They're high in soluble fiber, the type that helps lower cholesterol and keep blood sugar on an even keel. They're a surprising source of folic acid, that B vitamin women planning a family need to help reduce the risk of certain disabling birth defects. And potassium, the aid to blood pressure, is present in ample quantities. Unlike their carrot cousins, however, parsnips lack beta-carotene.

SELECTION AND STORAGE

Parsnips are root vegetables that are creamy yellow on the outside and white on the inside. They're available year-round in some markets but are easier to find in winter and early spring. The later parsnips are harvested, the sweeter they will taste, as the extra time and a frost help turn the starch into sugar.

Choose small- to medium-size parsnips; they'll be less fibrous and more tender. They shouldn't be "hairy" with rootlets or have obvious blemishes. The skin should be fairly smooth and firm, not flabby. If the greens are still attached, they should look fresh.

Before refrigerating, clip off any attached greens, so they won't drain moisture from the root. Parsnips stored in your crisper drawer in a loosely closed plastic bag will keep for a couple of weeks.

PREPARATION AND SERVING TIPS

Scrub parsnips well before cooking. (They're not for eating raw.) Trim both ends. As with carrots, cut ¼- to ½-inch off the top—the greens end—to avoid pesticide residues. Scrape or peel a thin layer of skin before or after cooking. If you do it after, they'll be sweeter and full of more nutrients.

Because parsnips tend to be top-heavy, they don't cook evenly. Get around this by slicing halfway down the fat end, or cut them in half crosswise and cook the fat tops first, adding the slender bottoms halfway through cooking. Steaming takes about 20 to 30 minutes. To speed cooking, cut them into chunks and steam them for 10 to 15 minutes.

For a change of pace, parsnips make a fine substitute for potatoes. They are a hearty accompaniment to beef and pork. Serve them whole, cut-up, or pureed like winter squash. For the latter, resist the urge to top with melted butter. Instead, try a dollop of nonfat yogurt. To bring out their sweetness, add ginger, dill weed, chervil, or nutmeg.

Parsnips are best in soups and stews. They help make a flavorful stock, or you can puree them for a flavorful thickener.

PARSNIPS, FRESH, COOKED
Serving Size: ½ cup sliced

Calories 63	Dietary Fiber ....3.3 g
Protein...........................1 g	Sodium.......................8 mg
Carbohydrate ....15.2 g	Vitamin C ....10 mg
Fat...............................<1 g	Folic Acid ....45 mcg
Saturated ....0 g	Manganese ....<1 mg
Cholesterol.................0 mg	Potassium ....287 mg

PASTA

Pasta has finally shed its fattening image, which was so undeserved. As a complex carbohydrate, it is digested slowly. And as for calories, at four per gram, pasta won't pack on pounds unless you eat platefuls or pile on creamy sauces. Eating healthy pasta dishes with a simple tomato sauce and lots of vegetables fights the fat in your diet by taking the place of fattier meat-based meals.

HEALTH BENEFITS

By glancing at the nutrients listed here, you can tell pasta is a health food. To help process its carbohydrates into energy, pasta even brings along its own B vitamins. Whole-wheat pasta is particularly rich in minerals and fiber, making it even more satisfying as a meal.

SELECTION AND STORAGE

Durum wheat, from which golden semolina pasta is made, is naturally higher in nutrients, including protein, than other types of wheat. But like white flour, durum flour is refined, so it's missing the nutritious bran and germ—the storehouses of valuable nutrients. More often than not, refined flours used to make pasta are enriched with three B vitamins—thiamin, riboflavin, and niacin—and iron, so most aren't nutritionally void. But if you're looking for the most nutritious type of pasta, whole wheat is superior. Its bran and germ are intact so it has many vitamins and minerals, including hard-to-get copper, magnesium, and zinc, which are missing in refined pasta. If you don't like the taste or chewiness of whole-wheat pasta, try mixing it with regular pasta, for at least half the benefit.

Dried pasta will keep in your cupboards for months, especially if transferred to airtight containers. Storing pasta in glass jars makes a pretty countertop display, but the exposure to light will destroy some of the B vitamins. So store it in a cool, dry place and away from light and air. When it comes to taste and texture, fresh pasta is better than dried pasta, but it's not practical for some people.

PREPARATION AND SERVING TIPS

Cooking pasta may seem simple, but note these finer points:

•Use a large pot of water—four to six quarts per pound of pasta. Pasta needs room to move or it gets sticky.

•Add a pinch of salt. It makes the water boil at a higher temperature, so the pasta cooks faster and the strands are less likely to stick together.

WHOLE-WHEAT SPAGHETTI, COOKED
Serving Size: 1 cup (2 oz uncooked)

Calories	174	Riboflavin	<1 mg
Fat	1 g	Niacin	1 mg
Saturated Fat	<1 g	Copper	<1 mg
Cholesterol	0 mg	Iron	2 mg
Carbohydrate	37 g	Magnesium	42 mg
Protein	8 g	Manganese	2 mg
Dietary Fiber	5 g	Phosphorus	124 mg
Sodium	4 mg	Zinc	1 mg
Thiamin	<1 mg		

ELBOW MACARONI, ENRICHED, COOKED
Serving Size: 1 cup (2 oz uncooked)

Calories	197	Thiamin	<1 mg
Fat	1 g	Riboflavin	<1 mg
Saturated Fat	<1 g	Niacin	2 mg
Cholesterol	0 mg	Copper	<1 mg
Carbohydrate	40 g	Iron	2 mg
Protein	7 g	Magnesium	25 mg
Dietary Fiber	1 g	Manganese	<1 mg
Sodium	1 mg	Zinc	1 mg

•After the water reaches a boil, add pasta gradually. This prevents the water from cooling down, which slows cooking.

•Don't overcook pasta, or the starch granules will absorb too much water, causing starch granules to rupture, making it very sticky. Pasta is best cooked al dente—tender but chewy. Five to ten minutes does it.

•Drain pasta immediately. Do not rinse; you'll lose valuable nutrients. To prevent sticking, immediately toss the pasta with a little sauce.

Pasta can fit into your fat-busting diet as long as you forget fat-laden Alfredo sauce or pesto swimming in oil. Try piping hot spaghetti topped with uncooked, chopped, homegrown tomatoes, fresh basil or arugula, and perhaps a light sprinkling of freshly grated Parmesan cheese. Or add your favorite vegetables to a low-fat marinara sauce for pasta primavera.

PEARS

Lucky for us, pears are in season all winter long, making it possible to enjoy their luscious sweetness for months.

HEALTH BENEFITS

The amount of fiber in other fruit pales of comparison to that in a pear. Much of it is insoluble, making the pear a natural laxative. Its gritty fiber may help prevent cancerous growths in the colon, too. Enough of the fiber is soluble so it provides the same stomach-filling, blood-sugar-blunting effect as other fruits. It also fights cholesterol by absorbing bile acids, forcing the body to make more from its blood cholesterol.

Pears provide a decent amount of copper, potassium, and vitamin C. They're also rich in boron, which is needed for proper functioning of calcium and magnesium. So pears may indirectly contribute to your bone health.

SELECTION AND STORAGE

The juicy Bartletts are the most common variety, fresh or canned. The d'Anjos are firmer and not quite as sweet as Bartletts. They are all-purpose pears, like Boscs, which have elongated necks and unusual dull-russet coloring. Bosc pears are crunchier than others, and they hold their shape when cooked. The runts, Seckels, are also a russet color, but they are sweeter than the others. Comices are the premier dessert pears—sweet and juicy. They are cultivated to have less fiber than other varieties. Asian pears look and crunch like apples but taste like pears.

Pears are picked before they're ripe. Left on the tree, they get mealy. Off the tree, the starch converts to sugar. You can't tell a ripe pear from its color; fragrance and touch are better indicators. Because a pear ripens from the inside out, once the outside seems perfect, the inside is on its way to rotting. So don't buy pears ripe; buy them firm but not rock hard. Ripen them at home in a ventilated paper bag, taking care not to pile them up or they'll bruise. Eat them when they just barely yield to pressure.

PREPARATION AND SERVING TIPS

To get a pear's full nutritional value, be sure to eat the skin. Of course, wash it well first. If still firm, pear slices work well in salads.

Of all the fruits, pears are arguably the best for cooking, becoming even more sweet and creamy when heated. For best results, cook only firm pears. The traditional method is poaching; try using wine or juice as the cooking liquid.

PEAR, FRESH
Serving Size: 1 medium

Calories 98	Dietary Fiber ....6 g
Fat.............................1 g	Sodium......................1 mg
Saturated Fat........0 g	Vitamin C ....7 mg
Cholesterol................0 mg	Copper.....................<1 mg
Carbohydrate ....25 g	Potassium ....208 mg
Protein.......................1 g	

PEAS

Green peas, like dried peas, are legumes, except they're eaten before they mature. As with all legumes, they're chock-full of nutrients and fat-fighting power, and they flaunt twice the protein of most vegetables, so they're the ideal substitute for fattier protein fare.

HEALTH BENEFITS

Their fiber, mostly insoluble, aids intestinal motility and may help lower cholesterol. Of the myriad nutrients peas provide, iron is particularly important since it's hard to find nonanimal foods with much of this blood-building nutrient.

Snow peas and other edible-podded peas don't contain the same amount of protein or nutrients green peas do. But they are rich in iron and vitamin C, which help maintain your immune system.

SELECTION AND STORAGE

Fresh green peas are only available in April and May. Choose firm, plump, bright-green pods.

Fresh snow peas—Chinese pea pods—are increasingly available year-round. Look for small, shiny, flat pods—they're the sweetest and most tender. Avoid cracked, overly large, or limp pods.

Sugar snap peas are edible pods like snow peas, but sweet like green peas. Select plump, bright-green pods.

GREEN PEAS, FRESH, COOKED
Serving Size: ½ cup

Calories	67	Thiamin	<1 mg
Fat	<1 g	Riboflavin	<1 mg
Saturated Fat	0 g	Niacin	2 mg
Cholesterol	0 mg	Vitamin B_6	<1 mg
Carbohydrate	13 g	Folic Acid	51 mcg
Protein	4 g	Copper	<1 mg
Dietary Fiber	2 g	Iron	1 mg
Sodium	2 mg	Magnesium	31 mg
Vitamin A	478 IU	Manganese	<1 mg
Vitamin C	11 mg	Potassium	217 mg

Fresh peas don't keep long. Because their sugar quickly turns to starch, the sooner you eat them the better.

When you can't get fresh peas, try frozen.

PREPARATION AND SERVING TIPS

Wash peas just before shelling and cooking. To shell, pinch off the ends, pull down the string on the inside, and pop out the peas. Steam for a very short time—six to eight minutes. They'll retain their flavor and more vitamin C if they retain their bright green color.

Snow peas just need washing and trimming before cooking. Sugar snap peas need the string removed from both sides. Snow peas are perfect in stir-fries; cook briefly—a minute or two. Try adding peas to pasta sauce or tuna casserole.

PEPPERS

Though a completely different plant, peppers serve a purpose similar to that of peppercorns: Peppers, especially the hot varieties, add flavor to otherwise bland low-fat dishes.

HEALTH BENEFITS

All peppers are rich in vitamins A and C, but red peppers are simply bursting with them. Besides being low in fat, peppers provide a decent amount of fiber as well.

Hot peppers' fire comes from capsaicin, which acts on pain receptors, not taste buds, in our mouths. Capsaicin predominates in the white membranes of peppers, imparting its "heat" to seeds as well. Whether hot peppers are good or bad for you is not clear. At least one study has found that capsaicin benefits people suffering from migraines. And it's been shown to act as an anticoagulant, perhaps preventing heart attacks and strokes. But capsaicin has confounded researchers by exhibiting both anticancer and procancer effects. And though you may think hot foods like peppers cause ulcers, they don't. There's no proof they even irritate existing ulcers.

Easy does it may be the best advice. If hot peppers bother you, cut back. It takes time to develop an affinity for and immunity to capsaicin's fire. Some people never do.

SELECTION AND STORAGE

Sweet peppers have no capsaicin, hence no heat. They do have a pleasant bite, though. Bell peppers are most common. Green peppers are simply red or yellow peppers that haven't ripened. As they mature, they turn various shades until they become completely red. Once ripe, they are more perishable, so they carry a premium price. But many people favor the milder taste that these varieties provide. Cubanelles, Italian frying peppers, are a bit more intense in flavor and are preferred for roasting or sautéing.

Hot chili peppers, or *chilies*—the Mexican word for peppers—are popular worldwide. Ripe red ones are usually hotter than green ones. Still, shape is a better indicator of heat than color. Rule of thumb: the smaller, the hotter.

For example, the poblano, or ancho, chile is fatter than most peppers and only mildly hot. Anaheim, or canned "green chilies," are also fairly mild. Jalapeño is a popular moderately hot pepper. Among the hottest are cayenne, serrano, and tiny, fiery habañero.

With all peppers, look for a glossy sheen and no shriveling, cracks, or soft spots. Bell peppers should feel heavy for their size, indicating fully developed walls.

Store sweet peppers in a plastic bag in your refrigerator's crisper drawer. Green ones stay firm for a week; other colors go soft in three or four days. Hot peppers do better refrigerated in a perforated paper bag.

PREPARATION AND SERVING TIPS

To cool the fire of hot peppers, cut away the inside white membrane and discard the seeds. Wash hands, utensils, and cutting boards with soap and water after handling them and use gloves to prevent the oils from irritating your hands. Avoid touching your eyes while handling peppers.

Bell peppers are delicious raw. They develop a stronger flavor when cooked; overcooked, they are bitter.

What to do if you swallow more than you can handle? Don't drink water; it spreads the fire around your mouth, making the heat more intolerable. Research from the Taste and Smell Clinic in Washington, D.C., has revealed that a dairy protein, casein, literally washes away capsaicin, quenching the inferno; so milk is your best bet. If you don't have any milk on hand, eat a slice of bread.

SWEET BELL PEPPER, FRESH
Serving Size: 1 pepper

Calories 18	Vitamin A
Fat...........................<1 g	green pepper .....392 IU
Saturated Fat.......<1 g	red pepper ......4,218 IU
Cholesterol.................0 mg	Vitamin C
Carbohydrate ....4 g	green pepper ....95 mg
Protein.......................1 g	red pepper ....141 mg
Dietary Fiber ....1 g	Iron..............................1 mg
Sodium.......................2 mg	

HOT CHILI PEPPER, FRESH
Serving Size: 1 pepper

Calories 18	Dietary Fiber ....na
Fat...........................<1 g	Sodium.......................3 mg
Saturated Fat.........0 g	Vitamin A
Cholesterol.................0 mg	green pepper .....346 IU
Carbohydrate ....4 g	red pepper ......4,838 IU
Protein.......................1 g	Vitamin C.................110 mg

PINEAPPLE

Although pineapples from Puerto Rico, Mexico, and elsewhere are cheaper, they aren't as juicy and flavorful as those from Hawaii. But all pineapples share the same fat-fighting characteristics—exceptionally sweet taste and high fiber content.

HEALTH BENEFITS

Serve pineapple for dessert and no one will complain about missing sweets. That's just one benefit of this delicacy. Moreover, its fiber will fill you up and might help keep you regular. Pineapple is also a sweet way to get your manganese, just one of many bone-strengthening minerals. One cup exceeds a day's recommended amount by 30 percent. You also get a decent amount of copper and thiamin, plus more than a third of your recommended vitamin C needs.

SELECTION AND STORAGE

When choosing pineapple, forget all the other tricks; let your nose be your guide. A ripe pineapple emits a sweet aroma from its base, except when cold. Color is not reliable; ripe pineapples vary in color by variety. Don't rely on plucking a leaf from the middle either. You can do this with all but the most unripe pineapples. And it can just as easily mean that it's rotten.

Choose a large pineapple that feels heavy for its size, indicating juiciness and a lot of pulp. The "eyes" should stand out. A ripe pineapple yields slightly when pressed.

— Pineapple

Once a pineapple is picked, it's as sweet as it will ever get. It does no good to let it "ripen" at home. It will only rot.

Preparation and Serving Tips

Tips on tackling a pineapple: Core it and peel the outside first, then cut into slices. Or cut into quarters, then scoop out the inside without peeling it at all. Refrigerate cut-up pieces.

Try fruit kabobs for a unique dessert: Alternate pineapple, strawberries, and other fruit on skewers. Or grill pineapple skewered with vegetables. Try pineapple on brown rice to give it zing—a great alternative to a meat-based dish.

Pineapple contains an enzyme—bromelain—that breaks down protein and is the reason why gelatin won't set when fresh pineapple is added. Use canned pineapple instead.

Pineapple, Fresh
Serving Size: 1 cup diced

Calories	77	Dietary Fiber	2 g
Fat	1 g	Sodium	1 mg
Saturated Fat	0 g	Vitamin C	24 mg
Cholesterol	0 mg	Thiamin	<1 mg
Carbohydrate	19 g	Copper	<1 mg
Protein	1 g	Manganese	3 mg

PLUMS

If you can't find a plum you like, you haven't tried hard enough. There are more than 200 varieties in the United States alone, some quite different than others. It pays to be adventurous and explore unfamiliar plums.

HEALTH BENEFITS

If you eat a couple of plums at a time, you'll get more than a fair dose of vitamins A and C, the B vitamin riboflavin, potassium, and fiber. None is in amounts to bowl you over, but they're important all the same.

SELECTION AND STORAGE

Plums are a summer pitted fruit, called a drupe, with a long season—May through October. Some plums cling to their pits and some have "free" stones.

Plums are generally either Japanese or European in origin. The Japanese types are usually superior for eating. Many European types are used for stewing, canning, or preserves or for turning into prunes.

Plum skins come in a rainbow of colors: red, purple, black, green, blue, and even yellow. Plum flesh is surprisingly colorful, too. It can be yellow, orange, green, or red.

There's no room here to chronicle the characteristics of every type of plum, but here are a few eating plums you're likely to encounter: Santa Rosa, Friar, Red Beauty, El Dorado, Greengage, and Kelsey.

—PLUMS

When choosing plums, look for plump fruit with a bright or deep color covered with a powdery "bloom"—its natural protection. If it yields to gentle palm pressure, it's ripe. If not, as long as it isn't rock hard, it will ripen at home. But it won't get sweeter, just softer. To ripen plums, place them in a loosely closed paper bag at room temperature. Check them frequently so they won't get shriveled or moldy. When slightly soft, refrigerate or eat them.

PREPARATION AND SERVING TIPS

Don't wash plums until you're ready to eat them, or you'll wash away the protective bloom. Like most fruits, they taste best at room temperature or just slightly cooler.

Although Japanese plums are best eaten out of hand, most European varieties are excellent for cooking. They're easy to pit—being freestone—and their firmer flesh holds together better. Try famous Damson or Beach plums for preserves.

A compote of plums and other fruits, such as apricots, is a traditional way to warm up your winter. Poach plum halves, skin on. Plum sauce is a treat on ice milk or mixed into yogurt.

PLUM, FRESH
Serving Size: 2 medium

Protein.....................1 g	Sodium.......................0 mg
Carbohydrate ....17 g	Vitamin A................426 IU
Fat............................<1 g	Vitamin C ....13 mg
Saturated..........<1 g	Riboflavin.................<1 mg
Cholesterol................0 mg	Potassium ....226 mg
Dietary Fiber ....2 g	

POPCORN

You may think popcorn seems undeserving of its own entry, but it's an important snack food and it can also be a healthful one, too. Popcorn is here as much for what it doesn't have as it is for what it does have. It fills you up—but not out.

HEALTH BENEFITS

What snack food do you know that provides fewer than 100 calories, no fat or sodium, and almost four grams of fiber in three cups? Only one—popcorn. The catch is that it must be air-popped popcorn with no added oil, butter, margarine, or salt. But don't knock it. It's chewy, tasty, and filling—everything a snack food should be.

Besides all that, popcorn provides protein. And you can't beat its fiber content, practically all of which is insoluble. Eat plenty of popcorn and with all the fiber you'll be less likely to suffer constipation. Plus your intestinal tract will also be less likely to harbor carcinogens and other toxins.

SELECTION AND STORAGE

Nutritionally, air-popping is the best method and the only way to avoid added oil. Not everyone is pleased with the taste, however. If you prefer popcorn with added oil, keep it minimal since the oil used is often a combination of saturated and *trans* fatty acids. Fortunately, some microwave popcorns have only half the fat and calories of regular popcorn. Some are as low as one gram of fat per serving, so check labels when you shop and try different brands to find one you like.

POPCORN, PLAIN, AIR-POPPED
Serving Size: 3 cups

Calories 93	Protein.......................3 g
Fat...............................1 g	Dietary Fiber ....4 g
Saturated Fat.......<1 g	Sodium.......................1 mg
Cholesterol.................0 mg	Magnesium ....32 mg
Carbohydrate ....19 g	Manganese ....<1 mg

What about ready-popped packaged popcorn? Most of them are loaded with fat, especially the popular cheese-flavored varieties—some get as much as three quarters of their calories from fat. So make sure you read the labels.

The good news in all of this is that no matter the variety, you still get the fiber bonus. Figure at least one gram per cup.

PREPARATION AND SERVING TIPS

You can do it the old-fashioned way and pop kernels in oil on the stove, but you'll add extra fat to your diet. If you refuse to air-pop, you're better off sticking with a light microwave popcorn.

If you want added flavor, try dusting popcorn with grated Parmesan cheese, which is tasty but adds some fat. Or flavor it with sprinkle-on butter substitute, garlic powder, or cinnamon.

POTATOES

Whoever coined the phrase "the lowly potato" certainly wasn't aware of its nutrient values. And anyone who still shuns the potato thinking it is fattening is missing out on a food tailor-made for the weight-conscious person; potatoes are extremely low in fat and very high in fiber.

HEALTH BENEFITS

Potatoes may seem high in calories, but they are nutrient-dense, meaning you receive many nutrients for those calories. The fiber is half soluble, half insoluble, so it helps to keep you regular and helps to lower cholesterol. And slowing down digestion helps to keep you full longer.

With the exception of vitamin A, a potato has just about every nutrient. Did you know potatoes are one of the richest sources of vitamin C? They are also very high in potassium, beating other potassium-rich foods. They are a good source of iron and copper, too. In fact, a potato a day is good for your heart, promoting normal blood-pressure levels.

SELECTION AND STORAGE

Boiling potatoes are red or white. They're small and round with thin skins that look waxy, signaling more moisture and less starch. Baking potatoes, also known as russets or Idahos, are large and long with brown, dry skin. Their lack of moisture makes them bake up fluffy. Long, white all-purpose potatoes are also known as Maine, Eastern, or California potatoes. New potatoes are not a variety of potato; they are simply small potatoes of any variety that have yet to mature. They look waxy with thin, undeveloped skins that are often partially rubbed away.

For all potatoes, choose those that are firm with no soft or dark spots. Pass over green-tinged potatoes; they contain toxic alkaloids, such as solanine. Also avoid potatoes that have started to sprout; they're old. If you buy potatoes in bags, open the bags right away and discard any that are rotting, because one bad potato can spoil a bagful.

Store potatoes in a location that is dry, cool, dark, and ventilated. Light triggers the production of toxic solanine. Too much moisture causes rotting. Don't refrigerate them, or the starch will convert to sugar. Don't store them with onions; both will go bad faster because of a gas the potatoes give off. Mature potatoes keep for weeks; new potatoes only a week.

Preparation and Serving Tips

Don't wash potatoes until you're ready to cook them. Scrub well with a vegetable brush under running water. Cut out sprout buds and bad spots. If the potato is green or too soft, throw it out.

Baking a potato takes an hour in a conventional oven, but only five minutes in a microwave (12 minutes for four potatoes). Prick the skin for a fluffier potato. If you are baking them in a conventional oven, it's inadvisable to wrap them in foil unless you like steamed, mushy potatoes. When boiling potatoes, keep them whole to reduce nutrient loss.

Remember, the potato itself is not fattening, but what you put on it may help expand your waist. Don't slather your potatoes in butter, margarine, sour cream, or cheese. Instead,

WHITE POTATO, FRESH, BAKED (WITH SKIN)
Serving Size: 1 large baking potato

Calories	220	Thiamin	<1 mg
Fat	<1 g	Niacin	3 mg
Saturated Fat	<1 g	Vitamin B$_6$	1 mg
Cholesterol	0 mg	Copper	1 mg
Carbohydrate	51 g	Iron	3 mg
Protein	5 g	Magnesium	55 mg
Dietary Fiber	4 g	Manganese	1 mg
Sodium	16 mg	Phosphorus	115 mg
Vitamin C	26 mg	Potassium	844 mg

eat them plain or top them with nonfat yogurt or nonfat sour cream, and sprinkle them with chopped dill, parsley, or scallions. Pile broccoli or other veggies on top for added nutrition, fiber, and satisfying bulk.

New potatoes are delicious boiled and drizzled lightly with olive oil, then dusted liberally with dill weed.

PRUNES

Though relatively high in calories for their size, prunes have a reputation as a dieter's friend. They add a powerful dose of fiber and some nutrients to your diet that are needed when you follow a lower-calorie meal plan.

HEALTH BENEFITS

Prunes are a sweet way to add fat-free laxative fiber to your diet. A single prune contains more than half a gram of fiber and more than one gram of sorbitol (a carbohydrate that our bodies do not absorb well). Large amounts of sorbitol can cause diarrhea. Prunes also contain the laxative, diphenylisatin. No wonder they prevent constipation. So snack away, just don't go overboard.

In contrast, prunes' reputation for being rich in iron doesn't hold true. In reality, they're a decent, but not spectacular, source. Prunes, however, get overlooked as a source of vitamin A, even though they provide more than ten percent of recommended levels. Potassium is another unexpected benefit you get from eating prunes, which is beneficial for blood pressure.

SELECTION AND STORAGE

When selecting prunes, look for well-sealed packages, such as those that are vacuum-sealed. After opening, seal the package or transfer the prunes to an airtight container or plastic bag. Stored in a cool, dry location or in the refrigerator, they'll keep for several months.

PRUNES, DRIED

Serving Size: 4 medium

Calories	80	Dietary Fiber	2 g
Fat	<1 g	Sodium	1 mg
Saturated Fat	0 g	Vitamin A	668 IU
Cholesterol	0 mg	Iron	1 mg
Carbohydrate	21 g	Potassium	250 mg
Protein	1 g		

PREPARATION AND SERVING TIPS

You can eat them out of the box, of course. They make a great portable fat-free snack. Combine them with dried apricots for a delightful mix of sweet and tangy flavors. Or mix them with nuts and seeds for a healthy trail mix. But watch out—the calories add up fast.

If you're not crazy about eating whole prunes, try prune bits in your baking. They'll add sweetness, flavor, and fiber to quick breads, snack bars, even pancakes. Better yet, for real fat-fighting success, puree eight ounces of pitted prunes and six tablespoons of hot water in a food processor for a great fat substitute to use in baked goods. Replace butter, margarine, shortening, or oil in your baked good recipes with half the amount of the prune puree. For example, if the recipe calls for one cup of butter, substitute a half cup of prune puree. Tightly covered, the prune puree will keep about one week in the refrigerator.

PUMPKIN

The pumpkin is an American original. Unfortunately, it seems most people associate pumpkins with Halloween or with Thanksgiving when it's enjoyed as pumpkin pie. Pumpkins, belonging to the squash family, have an understated taste that lends itself well to a variety of dishes. Besides, pumpkins make a great fat substitute in baking.

HEALTH BENEFITS

The distinctive bright orange color of pumpkin clearly indicates that it's an excellent source of that all-important antioxidant beta-carotene. Research shows that people who eat a meal plan rich in beta-carotene are less likely to develop certain cancers than those who fail to include beta-carotene–rich foods in their diet.

SELECTION AND STORAGE

Look for deep-orange pumpkins, free of cracks or soft spots. Though large pumpkins make the best jack-o'-lanterns, they tend to be tough and stringy, so they aren't the best for cooking—try smaller ones.

A whole pumpkin keeps well for up to a month, if stored in a cool, dry spot. Once cut, wrap the pumpkin and place it in the refrigerator; it should keep for about a week.

To prepare, wash off dirt, cut away the tough skin with a knife or a vegetable peeler, remove the seeds, then slice, dice, or cut the pulp into chunks. You might want to save the seeds;

PUMPKIN

Serving Size: ½ cup, mashed, cooked

Calories	102	Sodium	2 mg
Fat	<1 g	Vitamin A	1,320 IU
Saturated Fat	0 g	Niacin	1 mg
Cholesterol	0 mg	Vitamin C	6 mg
Carbohydrate	6 g	Calcium	18 mg
Protein	1 g	Potassium	181 mg
Dietary Fiber	1 g		

when toasted, they make a great snack. If you prefer something quicker and more simple, you can always opt for canned pumpkin. It's just as nutritious as fresh. For pies and purees, many say it tastes as good, if not better.

PREPARATION AND SERVING TIPS

Pumpkin pie is, without a doubt, Americans' favorite food use for pumpkin. But traditional preparation, with heavy cream and whole eggs, transforms a virtually fat-free food into one that's loaded with fat. Instead, substitute evaporated skim milk for the cream and use only one egg yolk for every two eggs the recipe calls for. You'll cut the fat to about 30 percent of calories, and we predict no one will know the difference.

Pumpkin can be used to make nutritious, delicious, and moist cookies. Likewise, you can substitute it for some of the fat in quick breads. How about pumpkin pancakes?

RASPBERRIES

This fragile, exquisite, and expensive berry is actually a member of the rose family. But there is nothing delicate about the fat-fighting fiber you get from this tiny fruit.

HEALTH BENEFITS

It's hard to believe a food could taste so good and be so good for you. But raspberries fit that description well. They are low in fat and calories and they are also a good source of fiber. Some of the fiber is insoluble, so it helps keep you regular. But much of it is found as pectin, a soluble fiber known to help lower blood cholesterol.

Besides being a good source of vitamin C—an antioxidant beneficial in the fight against cancer—raspberries contain a phytochemical, ellagic acid, believed to have anticancer properties.

SELECTION AND STORAGE

Because they are so fragile, choose and use raspberries with care and eat them right away. Look for berries that are brightly colored with no hulls attached. If the green hulls are still on the berries, they will be tart. Avoid any that look shriveled or have visible mold. They should be plump, firm, well shaped, and evenly colored, with no green. They should be packed in a single-layer container and have a clean, slightly sweet fragrance. When you get them home, don't expect to keep them around for long. It's best to eat them within a day.

RASPBERRIES

Serving Size: ½ cup

Calories	30	Dietary Fiber	2 g
Fat	<1 g	Sodium	0 mg
Saturated Fat	0 g	Niacin	1 mg
Cholesterol	0 mg	Vitamin C	39 mg
Carbohydrate	7 g	Manganese	1 mg
Protein	1 g		

PREPARATION AND SERVING TIPS

Just before serving, take chilled raspberries and rinse under cool water. For a low-fat dessert extraordinaire, top frozen sorbet or a slice of angel food cake with whole, chilled raspberries. Make a raspberry puree to pour generously (it's terrifically low in calories) over fruit salad, a slice of low-fat cake, pancakes, or waffles. If you're celebrating a special occasion, add chilled, ripe raspberries to your champagne. Raspberries also make a colorful, edible garnish.

Frozen raspberries in light syrup can be used to make a delicious frozen dessert. Puree the berries in a food processor first. Then, add skim milk and fresh lemon juice. Process all of the ingredients on low speed. Pour into an airtight container and freeze the mixture. Then process the frozen mixture in the food processor, and refreeze it. Enjoy.

RICE

Rice is the dietary backbone for over half the world's population. In Asian countries, each person consumes, on average, 200 to 400 pounds a year. Americans eat about 21 pounds per person, per year.

Rice is one reason why Asian diets are so low in fat. While Americans tend to view rice as a side dish to a meat-centered diet, Asians view rice as the focus of the meal. Increasing the amount of rice and decreasing the amount of meat served helps reduce fat intake.

HEALTH BENEFITS

Rice is an excellent source of complex carbohydrates and, if enriched, a good source of several B vitamins. It complements other protein alternatives well, particularly legumes. This makes it a good basis for a diet—a low-fat one at that. Using rice-based meals to replace meat will have a direct impact on your fat intake.

Brown rice provides three times the fiber of white rice. Research shows that rice bran, a small amount of which remains in brown rice, lowers cholesterol. It's also more slowly digested than the carbohydrate of processed white rice.

SELECTION AND STORAGE

Long-grain rice is the most popular variety in the United States. Cooked, the grains are fluffy and dry and separate easily. Medium-grain is popular in Latin-American cultures. Though fairly fluffy right after cooking, it clumps together

170   FOODS THAT MAKE YOU LOSE WEIGHT

once it cools. Short-grain, or glutinous rice, has nearly round grains with a high starch content. When cooked, it becomes moist and sticky so the grains clump together—perfect for eating with the chopsticks of Asian cultures.

Brown rice is the whole grain with only the outer husk removed. It is tan in color and has a chewy texture and a nutlike flavor. It is more perishable than white rice but keeps about six months—longer if refrigerated. White rice keeps almost indefinitely if stored in an airtight container in a cool, dark, dry place.

Expensive wild rice is not rice at all but a member of the grass family. It has a rich flavor and is higher in protein than other types of rice.

PREPARATION AND SERVING TIPS

If rice is bought from bins, as in Asia, it must be washed to remove dust and dirt. Packaged rice bought in the United States doesn't need to be washed. If it's fortified, rinsing washes away some of the B vitamins. However, it is a good

RICE, WHITE, LONG-GRAIN
Serving Size: ½ cup, cooked

Calories	131	Sodium	2 mg
Fat	<1 g	Iron	1 mg
Saturated Fat	<1 g	Manganese	1 mg
Cholesterol	0 mg	Niacin	2 mg
Carbohydrate	29 g	Pantothenic Acid	<1 mg
Protein	3 g	Thiamin	<1 mg
Dietary Fiber	1 g		

RICE, BROWN, LONG-GRAIN
Serving Size: ½ cup, cooked

Calories	109	Dietary Fiber	2 g
Fat	1 g	Sodium	5 mg
Saturated Fat	<1 g	Magnesium	42 mg
Cholesterol	0 mg	Manganese	1 mg
Carbohydrate	23 g	Niacin	2 mg
Protein	3 g		

idea to rinse imported rices. They may be dirty and are not enriched, so nutrients won't be washed away.

Cooking times for rice vary by variety and size of grain. Long-grain white rice takes about 20 minutes to cook. Long-grain brown rice takes longer—about 30 minutes. Short-grain brown rice takes about 40 minutes. Wild rice takes the longest—up to 50 minutes.

Water isn't the only cooking medium you can use to prepare rice. Try seasoned broth, fruit juice, or tomato juice for a change of pace. Dilute it to half strength with water. Be aware that when you add acid to the cooking water—as with juices—the rice takes longer to cook.

Though rice is often served alongside a main dish, it is better stir-fried and mixed with plenty of vegetables. Or try it as a cold salad with peas, red peppers, and a warm, low-fat vinaigrette dressing.

SOYBEANS

Though the United States is the world's largest grower of soybeans, more than half of the crop is exported. What a waste. Soybeans are one of the best plant sources of protein, nearly mimicking the perfect protein profile of milk. When used as a substitute for meat—which it does well because of its protein profile—a serving of soybeans can save you fat, especially saturated fat. You also get a fantastic fiber boost, both soluble and insoluble.

HEALTH BENEFITS

For fighting fat, you just can't beat soybeans for their versatility. Though surprisingly high in fat for a bean, it's mostly unsaturated. By lowering your blood level of LDL cholesterol (the "bad" cholesterol), soybeans' unsaturated fat is thought to reduce the risk of heart disease. Soybeans also happen to be one of the few plant sources of omega-3 fatty acids, which may aid in the battle against heart disease and cancer as well as arthritis.

Soybeans are loaded with a phytochemical called isoflavone, which may help combat breast tumors by dampening the ill effects of estrogen-like compounds. This fact may partly explain why Asian women, whose diets are typically rich in soybeans, are less likely to develop breast cancer than American women (soybeans are often poorly represented in American diets).

Most soy products contribute some calcium; tofu with calcium sulfate or calcium chloride is an even better source of the bone-building mineral.

Selection and Storage

When buying soybeans, make sure packaged bags are well-sealed. Check for insects if buying in bulk; pinholes indicate insect infestation. Store soybeans in an airtight container in a cool, dry place, up to a year.

Many people benefit from soy without ever seeing a bean; they simply rely on its many other incarnations. Textured vegetable protein (or TVP—a meat extender) is used in many soy-based products. Tofu is soy milk that's coagulated and pressed into blocks. Tempeh is fermented soybeans that are formed into a "cake." Miso is a combination of soybeans and barley or rice that is made into a strongly flavored, salty paste. Roasted soybeans, called soy nuts, are sold as snack food.

Tofu can be purchased in bulk, water-packed, or aseptically packaged. If you buy in bulk, follow safety precautions. Because it can harbor bacteria, tofu, except that which is aseptically packaged, must be refrigerated. So unless it's aseptically packaged, don't buy it if it's displayed unrefrigerated. At home, refrigerate unwrapped tofu immediately. For packaged tofu, check the "sell-by" date. Aseptically packaged tofu keeps without refrigeration for up to ten months, but refrigerate it once opened.

Because of their high fat content, all soy products are subject to rancidity. If you smell a rancid odor or see mold, throw the product out.

Preparation and Serving Tips

To prepare soybeans: Soak a half cup of soybeans overnight, add two cups boiling water, and simmer for two to two and

TOFU, "LITE" (1 PERCENT FAT)
Serving Size: 3 oz

Calories 35	Carbohydrate ....1 g
Fat.............................1 g	Protein.....................5 g
Saturated Fat.......<1 g	Dietary Fiber ....na
Cholesterol................0 mg	Sodium....................70 mg

SOYBEANS
Serving Size: ½ cup, cooked

Calories 149	Dietary Fiber ....5 g
Fat..............................8 g	Sodium......................1 mg
Saturated Fat.........1 g	Folic Acid ....46 mcg
Cholesterol................0 g	Iron...........................4 mg
Carbohydrate ....9 g	Calcium ....88 mg
Protein.....................14 g	Potassium ....443 mg

a half hours. To lessen soybean's gassy nature, throw out the soaking water, which contains indigestible carbohydrates, and cook them in fresh water.

The flavor of soybeans is bland, but that's their secret. The versatility of this culinary chameleon lies in its ability to take on the flavors of foods it's prepared with—enough so you forget you're not eating meat. Tempeh has the "meatiest" quality and works well as a meat substitute in stir-fry dishes. Miso works best as a taste enhancer, but if you're watching your salt intake, take it easy.

SPINACH

It seems Popeye had the right idea. Spinach is indeed a nutrition superstar, even a fairly good source of iron. It's loaded with vitamins and minerals, some of which are hard to find in other foods, and it's reasonably high in fiber—offering twice as much as most other cooking or salad greens. This helps you fight fat by filling you up with bulk.

HEALTH BENEFITS

Like other dark greens, spinach is an excellent source of beta-carotene, a powerful disease-fighting antioxidant that's been shown, among other things, to reduce the risk of developing cataracts. It fights heart disease and cancer as well.

Served raw, spinach is a good source of vitamin C, another powerful antioxidant. Overcook it, however, and you lose most of this important vitamin. Though spinach is rich in calcium, most of it is unavailable, because oxalic acid in spinach binds with calcium, preventing its absorption. When you cook spinach, it cooks down tremendously. Because cooking concentrates nutrients and fiber, a serving of cooked spinach gives you even more bang for your buck than a serving of raw.

SELECTION AND STORAGE

Two basic varieties of spinach are available—curly-leafed and smooth. Smooth is more popular, because curly-leafed is more difficult to rid of dirt that's buried in its folds.

Choose spinach with leaves that are crisp and dark green; avoid limp or yellowing leaves—an indication that the

SPINACH

Serving Size: 1 cup, raw

Calories	12	Sodium	44 mg
Fat	<1 g	Vitamin A	3,760 IU
Saturated Fat	0 g	Folic Acid	108 mcg
Cholesterol	0 mg	Vitamin C	16 mg
Carbohydrate	2 g	Iron	2 mg
Protein	2 g	Manganese	1 mg
Dietary Fiber	1 g	Potassium	312 mg

spinach is past its prime. Refrigerate unwashed spinach in a plastic bag; it'll keep for three to four days. If you wash it before you store it, the leaves have a tendency to deteriorate rapidly.

PREPARATION AND SERVING TIPS

Wash spinach leaves carefully and thoroughly, repeating the rinsing process two or three times. Even a speck of grit left behind can ruin an otherwise perfect dish.

Spinach is treasured for its versatility—it's tasty whether you serve it fresh or cooked. Either way, it can be added to dishes without adding extra fat. Warm spinach salads are a classic, but they are typically high in fat. For a tasty low-fat version, omit the bacon and egg yolks, and use mushrooms and garbanzo beans instead.

To cook spinach, simmer the leaves in a small amount of water until the leaves just begin to wilt, about five minutes. Top with lemon juice, seasoned vinegar, sautéed garlic, or a dash of nutmeg, and serve.

SQUASH

Because squash is actually the fruit of various members of the gourd family, it comes in a wide array of colors and sizes. Eating squash is particularly satisfying, because the bulk fills you up, allowing you to forgo fattier fare.

HEALTH BENEFITS

Though all varieties of squash are good nutrition choices, winter varieties tend to be more nutrient-dense. They generally contain much more beta-carotene and more of several B vitamins than tasty, summer squash. Butternut squash's beta-carotene content even rivals that of mangoes and cantaloupe. And that's a boon in the fight against cancer, heart disease, and cataracts.

SELECTION AND STORAGE

Despite seasonal growth patterns, most types of squash are available year-round, though winter squash is best from early fall to late winter. Summer varieties—with thin, edible skins and soft seeds—include chayote, yellow crookneck, and zucchini. Winter varieties—with dark skins too hard and thick to eat—include buttercup, butternut, calabaza, hubbard, spaghetti, and turban. Look for smaller squash that are brightly colored and free of spots, bruises, and mold.

The hard skin of winter squash serves as a barrier, allowing it to be stored a month or more in a dark, cool place. An added bonus: Beta-carotene content actually increases during storage. Summer squash only keeps for a few days; store it in your refrigerator's crisper drawer.

SQUASH, BUTTERNUT
Serving Size: ½ cup, cooked

Calories 41	Sodium......................4 mg
Fat............................<1 g	Vitamin A.............7,141 IU
Saturated Fat.........0 g	Niacin ....1 mg
Cholesterol.................0 mg	Pantothenic Acid......<1 mg
Carbohydrate ....11 g	Vitamin C ....15 mg
Protein.......................1 g	Calcium....................42 mg
Dietary Fiber ....3 g	Potassium ....290 mg

SQUASH, CROOKNECK
Serving Size: ½ cup, cooked

Calories 18	Dietary Fiber ....1 g
Fat............................<1 g	Sodium......................1 mg
Saturated Fat.......<1 g	Niacin ....1 mg
Cholesterol.................0 mg	Calcium....................24 mg
Carbohydrate ....4 g	Potassium ....173 mg
Protein.......................1 g	Manganese ....<1 mg

PREPARATION AND SERVING TIPS

After peeling (or not, if you like) and removing the seeds, winter squash can be baked, steamed, sautéed, or simmered. Summer squash, on the other hand, is cooked and eaten skin, seeds, and all.

Some savory seasoning suggestions for squash: allspice, cinnamon, curry, fennel, marjoram, nutmeg, sage, and tarragon.

STRAWBERRIES

Luscious strawberries are the most popular berries and are unique because they are the only fruit with seeds on the outside rather than on the inside. In season, strawberries need no extra sweeteners or toppings. They fight fat by eliminating the need for any other fatty sweet.

These delicate heart-shaped berries range in size from tiny wild varieties to larger cultivated ones. Generally, smaller varieties are more flavorful. Unfortunately, today's cultivated berries are bred with durability, not flavor, in mind. Still, in late spring and early summer, you can find superbly sweet strawberries at farmers' markets and green grocers.

HEALTH BENEFITS

As with all berries, they are a fabulous fiber find, with those little seeds providing insoluble fiber that keeps you regular and helps fend off digestive system woes, including hemorrhoids and varicose veins.

Most of all, strawberries are a super source of vitamin C, even better than oranges or grapefruit. Strawberries are also a good source of potassium. Because it keeps blood pressure in check, potassium may keep you from becoming a stroke statistic. Also, strawberries are one of the few fruits that contain ellagic acid, a phytochemical with cancer-fighting power.

SELECTION AND STORAGE

Look for strawberries that are ruby red, evenly colored, and plump, with fresh, green, leafy tops. Big does not translate into

STRAWBERRIES

Serving Size: 1 cup

Calories	45	Sodium	2 mg
Fat	1 g	Vitamin C	85 mg
Saturated Fat	0 g	Calcium	21 mg
Cholesterol	0 mg	Manganese	<1 mg
Carbohydrate	11 g	Pantothenic Acid	1 mg
Protein	1 g	Potassium	247 mg
Dietary Fiber	2 g		

juicy; in fact, smaller berries tend to be the sweetest. Avoid strawberries in containers with juice stains or berries packed tightly with plastic wrap. And walk on by if you notice soft, mushy, or moldy berries.

Strawberries spoil quickly. So it's best to buy them within a day of serving. Refrigerate unwashed strawberries loosely covered.

PREPARATION AND SERVING TIPS

Though they are superb served au naturel, strawberries can perk up any cereal, add pizzazz to any salad, or beef up pudding or gelatin. If strawberries become overripe, puree and add them to fruit drinks (strain the seeds, if you wish) or drizzle the puree over fruit salad for a low-fat dessert.

SWEET POTATOES

In some homes in the United States, sweet potatoes are only served at Thanksgiving, even though they are available year-round. Too bad. Sweet potatoes are one of the unsung heroes of a fat-fighting diet. For reasonable calories, you get a load of nutrients.

HEALTH BENEFITS

This starchy vegetable has bulk to keep your tummy full for hours. Yet its nutritional profile makes the calories worth it, especially since they are fat free. Its fiber alone is enough to make a sweet potato worth eating.

If a beta-carotene contest were held, sweet potatoes would tie carrots for first place. That may make them top-notch for fighting chronic diseases like cancer and heart disease. Sweet potatoes are also rich in potassium and vitamin C; a small potato provides almost half the daily allowance.

SELECTION AND STORAGE

Though often called a yam, a sweet potato is a different vegetable. True yams can only be found at ethnic markets. The sweet potatoes in supermarkets are either the moist, orange-fleshed type or the dry, yellow-fleshed variety that resemble baking potatoes in texture. The orange variety has a thicker skin, with bright orange flesh. It is much sweeter and moister than other varieties.

Look for potatoes that are small to medium in size, with smooth, unbruised skin. Avoid any with a white stringy

SWEET POTATOES
Serving Size: 1 potato (4 oz), baked

Calories	118	Pantothenic Acid	1 mg
Fat	<1 g	Vitamin B$_6$	<1 mg
Saturated Fat	0 g	Vitamin C	28 mg
Cholesterol	0 mg	Vitamin E	5 mg
Carbohydrate	28 g	Calcium	32 mg
Protein	2 g	Magnesium	23 mg
Dietary Fiber	2 g	Potassium	397 mg
Sodium	10 mg	Copper	<1 mg
Vitamin A	24,877 IU	Manganese	1 mg
Folic Acid	26 mcg		

"beard"—a sure sign the potato is overmature and probably tough.

Though sweet potatoes look hardy, they're actually quite fragile and spoil easily. Any cut or bruise on the surface quickly spreads, ruining the whole potato. Do not refrigerate them; it speeds up the deterioration.

PREPARATION AND SERVING TIPS

To cook sweet potatoes, boil unpeeled. Leaving the peel intact prevents excessive loss of precious nutrients and "locks" in its natural sweetness.

The dry, yellow variety can be used in just about any recipe that calls for white potatoes. The darker, sweeter varieties are typically served at Thanksgiving. Try them mashed, in a soufflé, or in traditional Southern sweet-potato pie. Resist candying them; it adds lots of unnecessary calories.

TOMATOES

Tomatoes are one of the most frequently consumed "vegetables" in the United States, whether raw, steamed, fried, stewed, crushed, pureed, or reduced to a sauce. Though thought of as a vegetable, tomatoes are botanically classified as fruits. They are also one of our best sources of vitamin C.

HEALTH BENEFITS

Tomatoes, it seems, are at the center of low-fat living. They naturally lend themselves to health-conscious cooking, being sweet yet low in calories and fat.

While not bursting at the seams with vitamins and minerals, tomatoes are indeed rich in vitamin C. This antioxidant plays a key role in maintaining a healthy immune system. They also contain beta-carotene and several other carotenoids that may have their own disease-preventing properties, particularly against heart disease and lung cancer. Tomatoes also offer a good dose of that possible stroke preventer, potassium.

SELECTION AND STORAGE

Red or yellow, tomatoes fall into three groups: cherry, plum, and round slicing tomatoes. Cherry tomatoes are bite-sized and perfectly round. Italian plum tomatoes are egg-shaped. Slicing tomatoes are large and round, perfect for sandwich slices. Beefsteaks are a popular variety.

Though available year-round, you may not want to eat what passes for fresh tomatoes in the wintertime. The best-tasting tomatoes are "vine-ripened," that is, they've been allowed to

TOMATOES
Serving Size: 1 tomato

Calories	24	Dietary Fiber	1 g
Fat	<1 g	Sodium	10 mg
Saturated Fat	0 g	Vitamin A	1,133 IU
Cholesterol	0 mg	Vitamin C	22 mg
Carbohydrate	5 g	Potassium	254 mg
Protein	1 g		

ripen on the vine, so they aren't made to ripen artificially. You may have to shop farmers' markets to find them. Moreover, there is no standard definition for the term "vine-ripened." Know your vendor before you trust the claim.

Look for tomatoes that are firm and well-shaped and have a noticeable fragrance. They should be heavy for their size and yield to slight pressure when gently squeezed.

A common mistake is to store tomatoes in the refrigerator. Cold temperatures ruin the taste and texture of a good tomato. Also, wait until you're just ready to serve them before you slice them; once cut, flavor fades.

PREPARATION AND SERVING TIPS

Salads seem more complete with a ripe, red tomato. Sliced tomatoes, served on a bed of radicchio or arugula, drizzled with a flavored vinaigrette or balsamic vinegar, and topped with fresh basil can't be beat. Chopped fresh tomatoes add flavor, color, and nutrition to soups, stews, and casseroles. They're superb on hot pasta.

WHEAT GERM

Wheat germ, a health-food basic, is the embryo of the wheat kernel. It is the portion of the wheat kernel that is removed when it is processed into refined flour. Wheat germ certainly deserves its reputation for being a powerhouse of nutrients, as its profile strikingly illustrates.

HEALTH BENEFITS

When you cut back on fat, you almost certainly cut back on the amount of meat you eat. When this happens, you may also be cutting back on important nutrients, too. Filling the void, though, is fat-fighting wheat germ. It provides a bevy of minerals, including all-important "meaty" iron and zinc.

Face it, wheat germ is a nutrition standout. It's one of the best sources of folic acid. That's good news, since the government is now recommending that all women of child-bearing age get sufficient amounts of this nutrient to prevent neural-tube birth defects. Newer research suggests that folic acid may help prevent heart disease. The fiber boost you get from wheat germ is phenomenal.

SELECTION AND STORAGE

Because of its fat content, wheat germ goes rancid easily, especially if it's raw. Fresh wheat germ should smell something like toasted nuts, not musty. Unopened, a sealed jar of wheat germ will keep about one year on the shelf. Always store opened wheat germ in the refrigerator in a tightly sealed container, where it'll keep up to nine months.

Wheat Germ

Serving Size: 1 oz, toasted

Calories	108	Thiamin	1 mg
Fat	3 g	Vitamin B_6	<1 mg
Saturated Fat	1 g	Vitamin E	4 mg
Cholesterol	0 mg	Calcium	13 mg
Carbohydrate	14 g	Copper	<1 mg
Protein	8 g	Iron	3 mg
Dietary Fiber	4 g	Magnesium	91 mg
Sodium	1 mg	Manganese	6 mg
Folic Acid	100 mcg	Phosphorus	325 mg
Pantothenic Acid	<1 mg	Potassium	269 mg
Riboflavin	<1 mg	Zinc	5 mg

PREPARATION AND SERVING TIPS

Wheat germ makes a nutritious and often undetectable addition to a myriad of dishes, including breads, pancakes, waffles, cookies, cereals, and milk shakes. It's a lower-fat alternative to granola that can be added to yogurt and cereals.

When adding wheat germ to baked goods or quick breads, you can replace one half to one cup of the flour with it. Because wheat germ tends to absorb moisture, you may want to add one to two tablespoons of water for every one-quarter cup of wheat germ you add to a recipe.

Yogurt, Nonfat

There was a time when yogurt eaters were considered "health nuts." Attitudes have changed. Today, yogurt is consumed by all sorts of people. Walk into any supermarket and you'll see a dizzying array of brands and flavors—and not all are so nutritious. Your best bet is to stick with nonfat yogurt.

Health Benefits

Yogurt may not be the miracle food some have claimed, but it certainly has a lot to offer. As a protein source, it is complete, so it can be used as the basis for meals, substituting for high-fat meats. It provides bone-building calcium in a dose as great as that from a glass of milk but can be digested more easily when live, active bacterial cultures are present. It also features riboflavin, vitamin B_{12}, and many minerals.

It's believed that the bacterial cultures used to make yogurt, *Lactobacillus bulgaricus* and *Streptococcus thermophilus*, carry their own health benefits. Research suggests that eating yogurt regularly helps boost immune function, warding off colds and possibly cancer. It's also thought that the friendly bacteria in yogurt help prevent and cure diarrhea. Another study has demonstrated that women plagued with chronic vaginal yeast infections found protection by eating a daily dose of bacteria-toting yogurt.

Selection and Storage

To ensure your carton is a welcome addition to a fat-busting diet, look for three traits when choosing a yogurt carton from the supermarket cold case. First, select one that's nonfat. Second, look for yogurt that contains live, active cultures. And third, it's best to choose plain, vanilla, lemon, or any yogurt without a jamlike fruit mixture added, which adds little nutrition but lots of calories. Also, check for a "sell-by" date on the carton. Refrigerated, yogurt will keep for up to ten days past that date.

Preparation and Serving Tips

Yogurt makes a great portable lunch, if kept cold. If you don't have access to a refrigerator, try freezing the carton; it will thaw in time for lunch. Yogurt also makes a delicious low-fat dessert. For either, try adding sliced berries, nuts, wheat germ, bananas, or low-fat granola. You can even top cereal with yogurt instead of milk.

Yogurt substitutes beautifully in recipes that call for high-fat ingredients like cream or sour cream. And yogurt is especially well-suited as a base for dips and salad dressings.

Yogurt, Nonfat, Vanilla
Serving Size: 8 oz

Calories	100	Pantothenic Acid	1 mg
Fat	0 g	Riboflavin	1 mg
Saturated Fat	0 g	Vitamin B_{12}	1 mcg
Cholesterol	5 mg	Calcium	389 mg
Carbohydrate	16 g	Magnesium	37 mg
Protein	12 g	Phosphorus	306 mg
Dietary Fiber	0 mg	Potassium	550 mg
Sodium	149 mg	Zinc	2 mg

– Index

Foods that Make You Lose Weight

Heart disease prevention *(continued)*
  mushrooms and, 128
  phytochemicals and, 8
  saturated fats and, 22–24
  vegetarian diet and, 7
  weight loss and, 5, 7
Hemorrhoids, 51, 62, 180
Hepatitis, 90
Homocysteine, 85, 131

Immune function, 25, 49, 188
Iron, sources of
  beets, 57
  dry beans, 54
  greens, cooking, 101
  herbs and spices, 106
  lentils, 115
  mushrooms, 127
  nuts and seeds, 131
  oats, 135
  pasta, 145
  peas, green, 150
  potatoes, 161
  prunes, 164
  spinach, 176
  wheat germ, 186
  whole-wheat bread, 65

Labels, food, 26–29
Lactobacillus bulgaricus, 188
Lactose intolerance, 122
LDL cholesterol, 24, 53, 93, 131, 173

Magnesium, sources of
  bananas, 49
  dry beans, 54
  kale, 109
  kiwifruit, 111
  mangoes, 117
  nuts and seeds, 131
  oats, 135
  pasta, 145
Manganese, 59, 101, 131, 135
Metabolic rate, 9, 17, 35
Migraine headaches, 89, 152
Monosodium glutamate, 127
Monounsaturated fats, 24, 26, 28
MyPyramid, 12, 13

Negative calorie effect, 20
Niacin, 65, 85, 127, 131, 145
Night blindness, 81
Norepinephrine, 17
Nutrition Facts. *See* Labels, food.

Obesity, 10
Omega-3 fatty acids, 7, 11, 26, 32, 89, 91, 131, 173
Omega-6 fatty acids, 26
Osteoporosis prevention
  boron and, 98
  calcium and, 100, 123

Pesticides, 42, 81, 91
Phytochemicals, sources of
  broccoli, 69
  brussels sprouts, 71
  cabbage, 77
  cauliflower, 83
  grapefruit, 96
  grapes, 98
  lemons and limes, 113
  raspberries, 168
  soybeans, 173
  strawberries, 180
Poisoning
  alkaloids and, 162
  contaminants in fish, 90–91
  wild mushrooms and, 129
Polyunsaturated fats, 24, 28
Potassium, sources of
  bananas, 49
  cabbage, 78
  cauliflower, 83
  dates, 87
  greens, cooking, 101
  kale, 109
  kiwifruit, 111
  melons, 119
  mushrooms, 127
  pears, 148
  potatoes, 161
  prunes, 164
  strawberries, 180
  sweet potatoes, 182
  tomatoes, 184
Prostaglandins, 21, 26

FOODS THAT MAKE YOU LOSE WEIGHT